D1621505

TREATING
SCHOOL-AGE CHILDREN

THE JOSSEY-BASS LIBRARY OF CURRENT CLINICAL TECHNIQUE

IRVIN D. YALOM, GENERAL EDITOR

NOW AVAILABLE

Treating Alcoholism
Stephanie Brown, Editor

Treating Schizophrenia
Sophia Vinogradov, Editor

Treating Women Molested in Childhood
Catherine Classen, Editor

Treating Depression
Ira D. Glick, Editor

Treating Eating Disorders
Joellen Werne, Editor

Treating Dissociative Identity Disorder
James L. Spira, Editor

Treating Couples
Hilda Kessler, Editor

Treating Adolescents
Hans Steiner, Editor

Treating the Elderly
Javaid I. Sheikh, Editor

Treating Sexual Disorders
Randolph S. Charlton, Editor

Treating Difficult Personality Disorders
Michael Rosenbluth, Editor

Treating Anxiety Disorders
Walton T. Roth, Editor

Treating the Psychological Consequences of HIV
Michael F. O'Connor, Editor

Treating Preschool Children
Hans Steiner, Editor

Treating School-Age Children
Hans Steiner, Editor

TREATING
SCHOOL-AGE CHILDREN

A VOLUME IN THE JOSSEY-BASS
LIBRARY OF CURRENT CLINICAL TECHNIQUE

Hans Steiner, EDITOR

Irvin D. Yalom, GENERAL EDITOR

Jossey-Bass Publishers • San Francisco

Substantial discounts on bulk quantities of Jossey-Bass books are available to corporations, professional associations, and other organizations. For details and discount information, contact the special sales department at Jossey-Bass Inc., Publishers (415) 433–1740; Fax (800) 605–2665.

Jossey-Bass Web address: http://www.josseybass.com

 Manufactured in the United States of America on Lyons Falls Turin Book. TCF This paper is acid-free and 100 percent totally chlorine-free.

Library of Congress Cataloging-in-Publication Data

Treating school-age children/Hans Steiner, editor; Irvin D. Yalom, general editor.
   p.   cm.—(A volume in the Jossey-Bass library of current clinical technique)
   ISBN 0-7879-0878-9 (paperback:alk. paper)
   1. Children—Diseases—Treatment. 2. School children—Diseases—
Treatment. I. Steiner, Hans, date. II. Yalom, Irvin D., date. III. Series: Jossey-
Bass library of current clinical technique.
RJ52.T74 1997
618.92—dc21
                                                   97-5198
                                                  CIP

FIRST EDITION
PB Printing 10 9 8 7 6 5 4 3 2

CONTENTS

974 70

FOREWORD

At a recent meeting of clinical practitioners, a senior practitioner declared that more change had occurred in his practice of psychotherapy in the past year than in the twenty preceding years. Nodding assent, the others all agreed.

And was that a good thing for their practice? A resounding "No!" Again, unanimous concurrence—too much interference from managed care; too much bureaucracy; too much paper work; too many limits set on fees, length, and format of therapy; too much competition from new psychotherapy professions.

Were these changes a good or a bad thing for the general public? Less unanimity on this question. Some pointed to recent positive developments. Psychotherapy was becoming more mainstream, more available, and more acceptable to larger segments of the American public. It was being subjected to closer scrutiny and accountability—uncomfortable for the practitioner but, if done properly, of potential benefit to the quality and efficiency of behavioral health care delivery.

But without dissent this discussion group agreed—and every aggregate of therapists would concur—that astounding changes are looming for our profession: changes in the reasons that clients request therapy; changes in the perception and practice of mental health care; changes in therapeutic theory and technique; and changes in the training, certification, and supervision of professional therapists.

From the perspective of the clientele, several important currents are apparent. A major development is the de-stigmatization of psychotherapy. No longer is psychotherapy invariably a hush-hush affair, laced with shame and conducted in offices with separate entrance and exit doors to prevent the uncomfortable possibility of clients meeting one another.

Today such shame and secrecy have been exploded. Television talk shows—Oprah, Geraldo, Donahue—have normalized

ix

psychopathology and psychotherapy by presenting a continuous public parade of dysfunctional human situations: hardly a day passes without television fare of confessions and audience interactions with deadbeat fathers, sex addicts, adult children of alcoholics, battering husbands and abused wives, drug dealers and substance abusers, food bingers and purgers, thieving children, abusing parents, victimized children suing parents.

The implications of such de-stigmatization have not been lost on professionals who no longer concentrate their efforts on the increasingly elusive analytically suitable neurotic patient. Clinics everywhere are dealing with a far broader spectrum of problem areas and must be prepared to offer help to substance abusers and their families, to patients with a wide variety of eating disorders, adult survivors of incest, victims and perpetrators of domestic abuse. No longer do trauma victims or substance abusers furtively seek counseling. Public awareness of the noxious long-term effects of trauma has been so sensitized that there is an increasing call for public counseling facilities and a growing demand, as well, for adequate counseling provisions in health care plans.

The mental health profession is changing as well. No longer is there such automatic adoration of lengthy "depth" psychotherapy where "deep" or "profound" is equated with a focus on the earliest years of the patient's life. The contemporary field is more pluralistic: many diverse approaches have proven therapeutically effective and the therapist of today is more apt to tailor the therapy to fit the particular clinical needs of each patient.

In past years there was an unproductive emphasis on territoriality and on the maintaining of hierarchy and status—with the more prestigious professions like psychiatry and doctoral-level psychology expending considerable energy toward excluding master's level therapists. But those battles belong more to the psychotherapists of yesterday; today there is a significant shift toward a more collaborative interdisciplinary climate.

Managed care and cost containment are driving some of these changes. The role of the psychiatrist has been particularly affected as cost efficiency has decreed that psychiatrists will less frequently deliver psychotherapy personally but, instead, limit their activities to supervision and to psychopharmacological treatment.

In its efforts to contain costs, managed care has asked therapists to deliver a briefer, focused therapy. But gradually managed care is realizing that the bulk of mental health treatment cost is consumed by inpatient care and that outpatient treatment, even long-term therapy, is not only salubrious for the patient but far less costly. Another looming change is that the field is turning more frequently toward the group therapies. How much longer can we ignore the many comparative research studies demonstrating that the group therapy format is equally or more effective than higher cost individual therapies?

Some of these cost-driven edicts may prove to be good for the patients; but many of the changes that issue from medical model mimicry—for example, efforts at extreme brevity and overly precise treatment plans and goals that are inappropriate to the therapy endeavor and provide only the illusion of efficiency—can hamper the therapeutic work. Consequently, it is of paramount importance that therapists gain control of their field and that managed care administrators not be permitted to dictate how psychotherapy or, for that matter, any other form of health care be conducted. That is one of the goals of this series of texts: to provide mental health professionals with such a deep grounding in theory and such a clear vision of effective therapeutic technique that they will be empowered to fight confidently for the highest standards of patient care.

The Jossey-Bass Library of Current Clinical Technique is directed and dedicated to the frontline therapist—to master's and doctoral-level clinicians who personally provide the great bulk of mental health care. The purpose of this entire series is to offer state-of-the-art instruction in treatment techniques for the most commonly encountered clinical conditions. Each volume offers a focused theoretical background as a foundation for practice and then dedicates itself to the practical task of what to do for the patient—how to assess, diagnose, and treat.

I have selected volume editors who are either nationally recognized experts or are rising young stars. In either case, they possess a comprehensive view of their specialty field and have selected leading therapists of a variety of persuasions to describe their therapeutic approaches.

Although all the contributors have incorporated the most recent and relevant clinical research in their chapters, the emphasis in these volumes is the practical technique of therapy. We shall offer specific therapeutic guidelines, and augment concrete suggestions with the liberal use of clinical vignettes and detailed case histories. Our intention is not to impress or to awe the reader, and not to add footnotes to arcane academic debates. Instead, each chapter is designed to communicate guidelines of immediate pragmatic value to the practicing clinician. In fact, the general editor, the volume editors, and the chapter contributors have all accepted our assignments for that very reason: a rare opportunity to make a significant, immediate, and concrete contribution to the lives of our patients.

Irvin D. Yalom, M.D.
Professor Emeritus of Psychiatry
Stanford University School of Medicine

INTRODUCTION

Hans Steiner

Ein Kind muss sich weit entwickelt haben, ehe es sich verstellen kann, viel gelernt haben, ehe es heucheln kann.
[A child must have developed considerably, before it is able to disguise, must have learned a lot, before it can be insincere.]

LUDWIG WITTGENSTEIN,
PERSONAL COMMUNICATION, 23RD NOVEMBER, 1994,
ST. GILES, CAMBRIDGE, ENGLAND

This book discusses state-of-the-art treatment of psychopathology as it appears in school-age children, those between six and twelve years old. This stage of life begins with the child's entry into school, one of life's major transitions, and ends in prepuberty, on the threshold of adolescence. Two other volumes in this series address the mental health needs of children younger than six and those of adolescents. As in our other volumes, all our recommendations are based on our clinical experience and research in the relevant fields, but we present the material in a clinical format to address the needs of the frontline clinician.

The ultimate challenge and reward for any mental health clinician is to enter the world of those we are helping in order to cure or soothe their distress. Such an enterprise is complicated enough in adults, as we attempt to distinguish manifestations of mental illness from ordinary reactions to stress and adversity, or in teenagers, with whom we must nimbly jump back and forth from adult to childlike functioning while braving the teeming energies of adolescent change.

In preparing to help school-age children, we encounter different and qualitatively new obstacles. Children's predominant mode of thought is more concrete. Connections that are obvious to us are not so for boys and girls between the ages of six and twelve, even if we point out and demonstrate them. For example, Piaget conducted well-known experiments that demonstrated children's limited ability to comprehend that different-shaped glasses can contain the identical amount of fluid, although such a thought is quite intuitive to the adolescent or adult mind. Another example of children's concrete mode of thought is their sense that death is not permanent; independent of their religious beliefs, children have only a slowly growing appreciation, not really entirely fixed in their minds, that death indeed means the permanent absence of someone.

If development proceeds as it should, children begin to conceal their innermost thoughts and desires, often from those about whom they care most, their families. As they encounter conflict between self-interest and group mandates, they deceive and even lie. What used to be an open stream of communication becomes a hidden brook bubbling under moss and branches. An essential step of socialization is taking place: children begin to develop a private life, a world of their own that no longer includes parents and those they are closest to. This process begins in the late preschool years and culminates in adolescence, but is clearly present in school-age children. You must reckon with the roadblocks this change creates for you.

As is usually true in life, the progress of socialization comes at a price: achieving privacy also means that one can misremember, repress, forget essentials, and even construct realities that did not exist. School-age children begin to develop private lives at unprecedented pace. Such a development is most likely driven by these newly acquired abilities to withhold information subtly from others with simple twists of reality and by using a completely new ability to in fact disguise information from themselves as well, especially if it is unpleasant. Erdelyi provides a wonderful example of such a "mental cleansing process." An elementary school girl was told a story about two Indian braves who were captured and who encountered other adversity, including the death of one of them. When the girl was asked to retell the story, she initially repeated all of the gory details. As time passed, however, she omitted more and more of the scary parts of the story.

The emotional content and flavor of childhood is also unique. If all goes well and according to expectations, the years just before puberty and adolescence seem quiet and uneventful, leading the classical psychoanalytic writers to pronounce this a "latency" period. Latency, in my opinion, is really a misnomer: a great deal is actually happening, but underneath a newly developing surface.

The new need for privacy has its most concrete manifestation in children's delight in developing secret societies and circles of friends that often have magical qualities and can only be entered with passwords. *The Secret Garden* describes such a process well, and has been for many years a favorite book for children in this age group, presumably because there is a natural resonance with age-appropriate tasks. Another manifestation of this interest in privacy is the fascination with mysteries, such as in *Pippi Longstocking* and the Nancy Drew stories. The world, children sense, is full of mysteries, but they can be understood and conquered if one is dogged in pursuit, cunning, and determined.

There are also forerunners of more familiar adult acquisitions and abilities during the school-age years. Children experience a new hunger for the unknown, a lust for exploration and learning. School is actually fun; children are excited to learn new things, expand their horizons, and freely share information acquired in the classroom and at home. Books about adventures in the wild continents of the earth are popular, as children try to enlarge the world beyond their homes and communities. Adventure and exploration also have more fantastic and unrealistic manifestations: heroes and heroines are popular, as are stories of gods warring for earth dominance. From Tarzan to Superman, from Wonder Woman to Brunnhilde, beings with superhuman qualities abound in fantasies and play. And when pressed, children may not be so certain that heroes and gods do not exist or at least did not at some point in our history. Often, such tales are placed in a space vernacular, as is *Star Trek*, because there appears at least some rationale for its assumptions: who can be certain that there are not other inhabited galaxies?

Children in this age group are able for the first time to have schemata of themselves, body and mind, and the word *self* begins to have a true meaning. Of course, with such progress come new problems: children now can start communicating distress through their bodies rather than through words; in fact, they can hide their mental distress behind bodily symptoms. A very common occurrence in this age group is the child's reporting of somatic symptoms when she has to face the teacher at school without homework or expects the return of a test with a failing grade. Headaches, stomachaches, and general feebleness appear as Mother comes to get the child up for school. Instead of saying, "I am worried about my grades and I don't want to face the teacher," the child is now able to say, "I feel sick."

Children between six and twelve are able to compare themselves to others and see how they themselves come up short. Such comparisons are often necessary in school, where grades are public and are some measure (albeit an inexact one) of one's standing in the class. Comparisons are also made about one's own and other children's popularity, and it is no coincidence that from this age on, peer nomination techniques can be used in research to gain very useful information about children's impressions of each other.

Children are also beginning to grapple with the problem of how to balance the needs of the self with the needs of a group, often practicing in their families first by refusing to do chores and such because, for example, they are too absorbed in a fascinating game. At school, we can observe the same phenomenon, as children compare the contents of lunch boxes, offer to trade or not as the case may be, and draw conclusions about the economic status of their friends on the basis of what is available to eat. In formalized activities, we can expect them to exercise considerable altruism with relatively minor supervision: much of what happens in Boy Scouts and Brownies is based on this realization.

Families, though, are still the solid bases on which children's lives and their mental health are founded, and if there is any quintessential period for family assessment and intervention, this is it. Parents, for the most part, are idealized and seen as all-powerful—a state much relished by all of us who have children, as it's only a short time before all this will change forever. Treatment in this age group can for the first time consistently use group approaches to achieve progress. Children still need some activity to absorb some of their energies in a session, but for the most part they can follow group process and be brought into it with relatively little encouragement.

The child is still supremely dependent on the family and has profound loyalty to them. You have to grapple with these loyalties as you expose intrafamilial conflict and try to get the child to express his dissatisfaction with family more openly.

Play therapy and individual psychotherapy can be particularly beneficial as children encounter family conflict with which they are not immediately able to deal. To feel angry and disappointed at the very person who takes care of you and supports you is a complex mental state, often leading to various maneuvers of appeasement and concealment. Because hidden conflict can continue to be a problem for the child, individual sessions without the parent present can be an important part of treatment.

As children's cognitive development begins to blossom, we gain new avenues into their private life and innermost conflicts. Children in this age group have the ability to act out what they feel by playing with toys or by drawing, sculpting, and painting. They also have the ability to step out of play and reflect on it, and can integrate the streams of thought and play to form new understandings, which are the basis of individual treatment. Play is highly symbolic, containing many metaphors and symbols for a child's life and mental states. Understanding such play and being able to respond to it effectively offer you powerful vehicles for understanding and change.

In order to enter the world of children, we need to prepare ourselves appropriately. Seeing patients and their families certainly helps, as does reading professional material, but we also recommend that you read the literary texts we refer to in the subsequent chapters and see a few current movies that deal with this age group. Such "immersion" techniques are a quicker way to bring us back in time, and they ready us to deal with the issues facing a child in this age group.

We also recommend that you revisit your own childhood to become aware of unfinished business, sore points, and leftover problems. Your own treatment can, of course, provide this awareness, but in addition we think it is quite effective to look at home movies and photographs. If possible, discussing your childhood with your parents is a rewarding exercise that quickly sensitizes you to the most salient issues outlined in our first chapter.

What is required of those of us who want to help school-age children? Perhaps the most outstanding characteristic is to be able to live on that edge between fantasy and reality, which is so powerfully important in children's lives. We need to be open to their reconstructions of this world, although we know that they are violating reality in significant ways.

To become effective, we need to suspend "big-people thinking" for a bit. For at least ten minutes a session, we need to be able to believe that Darth Vader could actually walk into the office, that Siegfried actually slayed a dragon, or that other universes are indeed possible. If we can do this successfully, we will enter a world in which magic can still be used to make things better.

We also need to be able to communicate in drawing, play, and words, and we need to switch between these channels at all times. Most of all, we need to be still and receptive, not to overwhelm what unfolds before us, which is a fragile web. We need to respect the child's experience. In our therapeutic encounters, time needs to be suspended. We have to be comfortable with children who retain their primary loyalty to their families, almost at all times, knowing that it is these very individuals who may create some of the child's symptoms. And we have to be able to forge an effective alliance with the child's parents as they are and will be for many more years, the great gyroscopes of socialization in our patient's lives.

The syndromes we encounter in this age group are reminiscent of classical psychopathology in adolescents and adults, but there are many qualitative differences that make the syndromes terra incognita and require special considerations and approaches. For example, depression in this age group is usually accompanied by many problems with hyperactivity, not by the psychomotor retardation we usually see in adults. Many depressed boys get referred for being naughty, not sad. As we will detail in Chapter One, treatment needs to incorporate techniques that are uniquely suited to this age group.

This book opens with an orienting chapter in which the authors summarize developmental information and lay out the principles of treatment and technique. What follows are a series of chapters on the most commonly encountered syndromes in childhood, their identification and treatment.

Anxiety-related disorders are quite common in school-age children; these disorders usually take the form of obsessions, compulsions, phobias, and trauma-related problems. Depression appears in full force, but in this age group depression usually has a strong component of behavior problems associated with it.

At this age, children's learning problems and oppositionality begin to crystallize into a diagnostic category that needs intervention at many levels to prevent poor outcome. Somatoform disorders appear for the first time, as does the child's ability to convert distress and conflict into symbolic physical symptoms. Drawing the distinction between these two forms of "speaking with one's body" can be difficult and troublesome. Pain and its management are major issues for school-age children, as certain chronic physical illnesses begin to appear and exact their toll on young lives. Child abuse is a critical issue for children of all ages; we must explore approaches to identifying, managing, and treating abuse and its consequences appropriately. And problems with food, weight, body image, and eating can make their first clinical appearance.

As in our previous volume on adolescents, we have followed the principle of presenting you with specific recommendations for treatment that are based on research (preferably our own data, as they are the most familiar and accessible to us). Once again, the chapter authors are experts in their respective fields. All of them either work here at Stanford or are graduates of our program and have accepted positions in other medical schools. All the authors have developed the particular style of practice taught in our program, which makes this volume cohesive and yet comprehensive.

ACKNOWLEDGMENTS

As always, we need to thank individuals who have helped us in the process of learning about treatment and in writing this book. First and foremost, my thanks go to Frances and Ted Geballe, who in their tireless fashion have taken it upon themselves to help many children, some in very personal direct ways, others through their support of our programs in school screening and intervention. Secondly, as always, we have to thank our patients and their parents, who have been our greatest teachers. Finally, I would like to thank the staff of the Roth Unit at Children's Hospital at Stanford, who for two decades have supported all of us so diligently and superbly in our efforts to deal with even the most difficult situations.

Thanks also to Marsha Wallace for help with the editing and production of drafts as well as the coordination for this endeavor; and once again to Alan Rinzler, for providing us yet another chance for personal growth.

NOTES

P. xiv, *Piaget conducted well-known experiments:* Elkind, D. (1977). *Children and adolescents: Interpretive essays on Jean Piaget.* New York: Oxford University Press; Ginsburg, H., & Opper, S. (1969). *Piaget's theory of intellectual development.* Englewood Cliffs, NJ: Prentice Hall.

P. xiv, *Erdelyi provides a wonderful example of such a "mental cleansing process":* Erdelyi, M. H. (1990). Repression, reconstruction, and defense: History and integration of the psychoanalytic and experimental frameworks. In Singer, J. L. (Ed.), *Repression and dissociation* (pp. 1–31). Chicago: University of Chicago Press.

P. xv, *manifestation in children's delight in developing secret societies and circles of friends:* Donner, J. (Producer) & Bergman, I. (Director). (1982). *Fanny and Alexander* [Film]. Nelson Entertainment.

P. xv, The Secret Garden *describes such a process well:* Burnette, F. H. (1962). *The secret garden.* Philadelphia: Lippincott. (Original work published 1911)

P. xv, *the fascination with mysteries . . . Nancy Drew stories:* Lindgren, A. (1950). *Pippi Longstocking.* New York: Viking Penguin; Keene, C. (1996). *Nancy Drew files no. 115: Running into trouble.* New York: Pocket Books.; also see the Hardy Boys mystery book series by Dixon, F. W. (1967). New York: Grosset & Dunlap.

P. xv, *Books about adventures in the wild continents:* Nordhoff, C., & Hall, J. N. (1932). *Mutiny on the Bounty.* New York: Little, Brown.

P. xv, *heroes and heroines are popular:* Burroughs, E. R. (1914). *Tarzan of the apes.* Chicago: A. C. McClurgh; Spann, M., & Leopold, W. F. (1953). *Die Nibelungen.* Lexington, MA: Heath. (Original work published 1250); Harris, J. (1992). *Wonderwoman and Superman.* Oxford: Oxford University Press.

P. xv, *tales are placed in a space vernacular, as is Star Trek:* Roddenberry, G. (Producer) & Wilson, R. (Director). (1980). *Star trek, the motion picture* [Film]. Paramount Pictures.

P. xviii, *that Darth Vader could actually walk into the office:* Lucas, G. (Screenwriter), Kershner, I. (Director), & Kurtz, G. (Producer). (1984). *The empire strikes back* [Film]. Twentieth Century Fox; a Lucasfilm Limited Production.

P. xviii, *that Siegfried actually slayed a dragon:* Hofler, O. (1978). *Siegfried, Arminius und der Nibelungenhort.* Wien: Verlag der Osterreichischen Akademie der Wissenschaften.

P. xviii, *enter a world . . . make things better:* Manlove, C. N. (1942). *The Chronicles of Narnia: The patterning of a fantastic world.* New York: Twayne.

Für Judith Königin von Narnia und
Kaiserin der Versteckten Villa

TREATING
SCHOOL-AGE CHILDREN

I

GENERAL PRINCIPLES AND TREATMENT

Richard J. Shaw and S. Shirley Feldman

During middle childhood, children experience remarkable developments in their social, academic, and cognitive abilities. This "school-age" period begins at six to seven years of age and ends with the transition to adolescence. Although Freud referred to this period as the phase of latency, it is, in fact, anything but quiescent. Over a very short period of time, a young child learning letters will soon be reading novels. Children enter this period counting on their fingers and leave it being able to calculate complicated mathematical problems in their heads. These academic achievements become a source of pride to the child and a major concern for parents. Children also become increasingly autonomous as they develop important peer and social relationships outside the family. These relationships, in turn, become an important influence on children's social and moral development.

Clinicians who work with school-age children are most successful if they understand the developmental issues unique to the age group and are aware of the typical range of behaviors, conflicts, and anxieties seen in the school-age child.

In this chapter we review the academic, cognitive, and social developments of the school-age child, and discuss how these developments affect self-esteem and social interactions. We then look at the important consequences of developmental problems in each domain. It is important to keep in mind that when children do not successfully negotiate the developmental tasks of this period they are likely to suffer from deficits in self-esteem and to experience subsequent difficulties during adolescence. We conclude the chapter with an overview of the principles of treating the school-age child.

ACADEMIC AND COGNITIVE DEVELOPMENT

Maturation refers to the sequential emergence of physical, cognitive, and motor abilities. These abilities enable a child to acquire new academic skills. Maturation implies that development proceeds along a biologically determined trajectory, provided that an appropriate environment exists to support the emergence of new characteristics.

Between the ages of five and seven years, and following a maturational timetable, the child's brain undergoes significant changes in the patterns of electrical activity, and the surface area of the brain's frontal lobes expands dramatically. A fatty sheath of cells called myelin begins to cover individual neurons in the brain. Myelin enables faster transmission of nerve impulses, and changes the interconnections in different areas of the brain. Researchers believe that these changes allow the frontal lobes to coordinate activities in other areas of the brain, resulting in increased capacity for focused attention, memory, planning, and self-reflection. This biological maturation enables the school-age child to develop his or her academic and cognitive skills.

Failure in brain maturation, as seen in children with cerebral palsy, or neuronal damage resulting from brain infections or head injuries, may lead to delays in development or actual loss of already developed abilities.

Cognitive Development

Although cognitive development in middle childhood includes many important changes, our focus here will be on attention and memory. These two areas affect how children come to think in a clear and effective way.

Attention. The ability to concentrate on tasks and pay attention to new material improves significantly in school-age children. By age six, the typical child can sit still for only ten to fifteen minutes, with adult supervision necessary to keep the child's attention focused. By age twelve, the typical child can sit still and concentrate for up to forty-five minutes and can work independently. Children develop the ability to block out distracting or irrelevant stimuli, and they become increasingly more flexible in being able to shift their attention from one topic to another. These capacities are essential for effective learning in the classroom. Children diagnosed with Attention Deficit Hyperactivity Disorder have such frequent disruptions in attention that succeeding in school becomes quite difficult for them. Boys in particular seem to be susceptible to disorders of attention.

Memory. School-age children demonstrate significant increases in their memory capacity. Children in this age group also become capable of using different strategies to remember things. For example, mnemonic strategies such as *rehearsal* and *memory organization* (rearranging material into meaningful clusters to facilitate recall) improve memory capacity. Another remarkable change is children's growing ability to focus on one activity without losing information from other unrelated activities and experiences.

Why are these new abilities important? Memory is not only necessary when children learn to read (for example, remembering the difference between a *b* and a *d*, or a *p* and a *q*) but is also essential for the acquisition of new vocabulary. As memory improves, children are increasingly able to remember instructions and directions and to act on them independently without the need for supervision. The ability to learn independently creates many opportunities for both the school-age child and the teachers of school-age children.

Piaget: Concrete Operations. Jean Piaget, a Swiss child psychologist, made important contributions to our understanding of the way children think and acquire knowledge. He noted that children in this age group learn in a qualitatively different way than do younger children. It is not simply that they know more facts or have longer attention spans and faster processing times but also that they reason and understand the world in a different manner than younger children. Piaget termed this new level of thinking and information processing the phase of *concrete operations.* School-age children can order, separate, and transform objects in their mind—but only with tangible, known objects. Children can reason about school, dogs, and baseball, but not about such abstract issues as justice, responsibility, and civil rights. The following list summarizes the characteristics of Piaget's concrete operations stage of cognitive development.

Piaget's Stages of Cognitive Development: Concrete Operations

- Children master the concept of *conservation:* even though objects may change in shape or form, children now recognize that key properties remain invariant. For example, a child will be able to understand that the quantity of water in a glass remains the same, even if it is poured into a different shaped container, or whether it is in the form of ice or water.

- Children understand the concept of *reversibility:* for example, in arithmetical problems that 7 x 3 = 21, and that 21 ÷ 3 = 7.

- Children understand relational terms: for example, the concepts of bigger than, or less than, in relation to physical quantities. This concept is essential for an understanding of numbers.

- Children develop the ability to attend to external information from multiple sources and to integrate different points of view. They become increasingly able to understand and accept other people's perspectives, signifying a decline in *egocentrism,* which is characteristic of younger children.

- Children are increasingly able to follow rules and regulations.

- Children develop the capacity for moral reasoning and can differentiate *intentional* misdeeds from *accidental* ones.

By understanding Piaget's stages of cognitive development, we can better understand the social and academic achievements possible at various ages. For example, in middle childhood, concrete operations facilitate the development of increasingly complex social skills as well as a greater ability to communicate and negotiate. School-age children develop the capacity to think about how they are perceived and understand that people may think in one way but act in another. They also develop the capacity for moral reasoning, which helps them appreciate the concept of rules in play and sets the stage for increased social cooperation in their peer relationships.

Academic Skills Development

The five- or six-year-old child starting school faces many new situations that require significant adaptation. The six-year-old must be able to tolerate separation from home for three to four hours per day, take instruction from teachers, inhibit his or her own wishes (such as when moving around during classes or speaking out of turn), and participate as a member of a group. Mastering these behavioral and social skills, as well as the fundamentals of reading, writing, and arithmetic, occupies the first few years of schooling.

Mastery of the "three R's" enables children to develop a feeling of competence and to move along the path of literacy essential for functioning in the modern world. However, classroom learning also provides the opportunity for children to compare themselves to others, which creates the possibility for damage to self-esteem. For example, a child at the bottom of a gifted class may not feel proud of his or her exceptional abilities, and being pushed too far in such a class may damage the child's self-esteem.

Although formal education in most cultures focuses on teaching children to read and write, many children experience difficulties with this process, despite normal intelligence. The ability to read requires general skills referred to as *decoding*, or the association of written characters with spoken sounds, and *comprehension*, the ability to assign meaning to the written text. Although preschool-age children master basic rules of grammar in their comprehension and speech, the ability to understand complex grammar and the connection between written and spoken words does not develop until the school years. School-age children come to understand that words may have both a literal and non-literal meaning and develop the capacity to use words in a play-ful and humorous manner, as in the following example.

> *Girl:* Knock, knock!
> *Boy:* Who's there?
> *Girl:* Isabel.
> *Boy:* Isabel who?
> *Girl:* Is a bell necessary on a bicycle?

By the sixth grade, the child's everyday language is compara-ble to that of adults, and subsequent changes involve primarily elaboration of vocabulary. In fact, much of the language of American television is pitched at a sixth-grade level. Whereas changes in thinking, as described by Piaget, involve qualitative changes, the changes in language are more gradual and quanti-tative.

Influences Affecting Academic Development

Although what children learn may vary tremendously from cul-ture to culture, it appears that the developmental sequence of middle childhood is similar across all cultures. The attainment of the skills described by Piaget occurs whether the child is raised on a rural African farm or in a large American city. How a child applies these skills and develops his academic potential, however, depends on a host of factors ranging from temperament to such environmental factors as culture, family, and school.

Cognitive Style Influences. Jerome Kagan noted that children may have very different temperamental styles when it comes to learning. For example, impulsive children tend to respond quickly and without reflection, often giving the wrong answer; by contrast, reflective children respond slowly and more thoughtfully. Understanding a child's cognitive style can be an important part of devising strategies to assist the child; for example, an impulsive child can be taught to pause before responding to questions. Paying attention to learning styles will help enhance the child's learning, which in turn promotes self-esteem and at the same time helps teachers provide effective group instruction without interruption.

Family Influences. Children whose parents take an active interest in their school performance are more likely to have high levels of academic achievement. This finding is particularly notable in Asian immigrant families whose children, despite social and economic disadvantages, frequently excel academically. By contrast, families who show indifference to their children's school activities may promote children's feelings of irrelevance and inadequacy. These findings have led educators to encourage, and in some cases require, parent participation in such programs as Head Start and in many elementary classrooms.

Peer Influences. Peer groups can also affect the academic performance of school-age children. Many types of peer groups exist: some value athletic prowess; others value being tough, having a good time, or being successful in school. Those peer groups that devalue academic achievement undermine the school's attempts to foster educational competence, and these group members typically do poorly academically. Peer groups can, however, also have positive effects on learning. Educators frequently use peer groups to promote interest in academic activities and school involvement.

School Atmosphere. School atmosphere can influence a child's interest in academic development. Schools that demonstrate a strong commitment to and expectation of academic achievement produce more successful students. The attitudes of the teachers and their skill in managing classroom behavior also have an impact on students. A classroom atmosphere that emphasizes praise and positive incentives more effectively nurtures students than one that relies on punishment. Elementary school children respond best to teachers who are warm but who demand high standards of conduct and achievement.

Clinical Problems Involving Cognitive Development

The previous section reviewed some aspects of academic and cognitive development in school-age children, and the factors which influence this development. In this section we consider some common clinical syndromes that result from problems in different areas of academic and cognitive development.

Attention Deficit Hyperactivity Disorder. Most schools teach in a way that requires children to sit still in a classroom and pay attention to written and spoken material. However, a significant proportion of school-age children, boys more commonly than girls, have difficulty focusing, controlling their impulses, and sitting still. These children often exhibit impulsive, moody behavior and show difficulties in both sustaining attention and in shifting focused attention from one topic to another. Mark, a six-year-old boy, is an example of one such child.

MARK

Described by his parents as an active and energetic child from birth, Mark was referred for evaluation by his teachers. At school, Mark was unable to stay in his chair for longer than five minutes without bothering his classmates and fidgeting. He would dart around the room, apparently unable to focus on anything for more than a few minutes. His work was disorganized and generally incomplete. If a teacher asked him a question, Mark would blurt out a response before the teacher had finished speaking, giving the impression that he was not even listening. He was impulsive in every respect, constantly on the go and rushing from one thing to another.

Viewed as uncooperative and disruptive, children like Mark encounter frequent criticism from teachers and parents as well as rejection from their peers. These social difficulties, combined with concomitant academic problems, frequently lead to feelings of low self-esteem.

Children diagnosed with Attention Deficit Hyperactivity Disorder make up a significant proportion of those referred for psychiatric treatment. However, debate continues about how to manage this disorder. One school of thought claims that the disorder is related to biological or environmental factors and should be treated with specific behavioral and pharmacological treatments, most commonly stimulant medications (such as Ritalin). Others argue that the symptoms are a manifestation of temperamental differences and that treatment with stimulants is an attempt at social control. Instead, they recommend reform of the educational system to better serve children with differing cognitive styles. Please refer to Chapter Four for a more extended discussion.

Learning Disabilities. Many children with normal intelligence have problems with reading and writing. These children are frequently but erroneously assumed to be mentally retarded, emotionally disturbed, or lacking in motivation. Children with dyslexia, for example, have problems with reading and spelling; they may see letters upside down or reversed, and may be unable to correctly reproduce the exact sequencing of language sounds. Children with learning disabilities frequently manifest accompanying psychological and behavioral problems that increase as they encounter negative evaluations, criticism, and rejection.

It is not clear why children develop learning disorders. Genetic factors, toxic events during pregnancy and early childhood, and environmental and social stressors have been implicated. Although children do not generally outgrow learning disabilities, early intervention (typically involving teaching outside the regular classroom) can reduce the potentially adverse effects on academic and social development.

PEER AND PARENT RELATIONSHIPS

During middle childhood a child's relationships with peers and with parents become more complex. Changes in the child's mode of thinking begin to affect relationships with other people, and similarly, these relationships with other people may influence the development of the child's self-concept. A greater awareness of self and of other's opinions, and a sense of right, wrong, and fairness, all make relationships and situations take on new meanings. How well a child learns to negotiate interpersonal relationships affects his or her self-esteem and sense of social competence.

Children's Play

Most children begin to spend more time with peers during middle childhood, and the nature of these interactions shifts to reflect developing cognitive skills. School-age children show an increasing interest in joint play, and friendships develop based on shared experiences. Peer groups are usually segregated by sex, based on the preference for different activities and different styles of interaction. Girls tend to have fewer but more intimate friends compared with their male counterparts. Boys appear to engage in more aggressive and competitive play, whereas girls engage in more cooperative and empathic interactions.

Developments in thinking, especially the enhanced ability to take account of another person's perspective, enable school-age children to engage in rule-based play. In such activities, children must agree on the rules of play ahead of time, balance individual desires and impulses with the need to conform to social rules, and learn to negotiate and resolve conflicts during games. Their success in negotiating play will extend to success in working with larger groups in many different situations.

Competitive sports organized by adults, such as Little League baseball or soccer, emphasize (in principle at least) the importance of sportsmanship and teamwork. Success in this arena not only leads to a child's feeling of acceptance by peers but also contributes to the development of his or her self-esteem. Conversely, the child may be exposed to the hazards of parents or coaches who are overinvested in "winning at all costs," and may experience internal or external pressure to deceive or cheat. The less-than-gifted athlete may also feel inadequate compared with peers and may experience rejection when not selected to play on the team.

Moral Development

During middle childhood, children develop an increasingly sophisticated sense of right and wrong; they come to understand the concept of rules as negotiated agreements based on the principles of justice and fairness, particularly regarding the treatment of individuals. This is also the age at which children learn a body of conventions and customs regarding manners and appropriate social conduct.

Debate abounds regarding theories of moral development. Psychoanalytic theories suggest that young children model themselves on their parents' standards of conduct, initially with the goal of avoiding punishment. During the school-age period, children take greater responsibility for their behavior and accept the values of their parents as their own. As external values become internalized, they become part of the child's conscience, which plays an increasingly important role in regulating behavior and in providing feelings of self-approval. Thus the emergence of conscience plays a pivotal role in self-esteem as well as in morality.

Lawrence Kohlberg suggested a theory of moral knowledge that is based on developmental changes in thinking. In the preschool and early school years, the desire to avoid punishment motivates much of the child's behavior. During middle childhood years (and for some years thereafter), the child strives for social approval from others and begins to show respect for authority. The child is increasingly able to acknowledge other people's perspectives and take into account intentionality in judging violations and misconduct.

Peer Acceptance

A major goal of this period is for the child to develop feelings of social competence and acceptance. Children who are attractive, intelligent, cooperative, friendly, and sensitive to the needs of others are likely to find social acceptance with their peers. When entering a new peer group, popular children take time to see the frame of reference of the new group and tend not to draw attention to themselves. These children generally have high self-esteem and evaluate themselves as being both effective and competent.

Children who are not well accepted by their peers tend to fall into two main categories: those who are aggressive and those who are withdrawn. *Aggressive* children paradoxically tend to deflect feelings of criticism; they have high self-esteem and see themselves as competent. Nonetheless, their aggressive behavior results in rejection in new peer groups. *Withdrawn* children, by contrast, have low self-esteem and describe themselves as being incompetent and low in self-efficacy.

Parents play an important role in their child's ability to develop peer relationships by promoting empathy, consideration, social responsibility, and self-restraint. A coercive family atmosphere will likely produce children who are more aggressive and coercive with their peers and more likely to show behavioral disorders in the classroom. Similarly, parents who are not effective in setting limits on their children's behavior may foster the development of children unable to conform to social norms.

These children are consequently also more likely to be rejected by their peers.

Significantly, peer rejection tends to predict school-related difficulties, such as truancy and academic failure, as well as delinquency, substance abuse, depression, and suicide. Children who do not manage to develop satisfactory peer relationships have a much greater risk of maladjustment and problems in later life.

Relationships with Parents

Parents play many different roles in a child's life. On a very fundamental level, parents provide material resources, including food, shelter, and financial support for education, medical care, and recreational activities. Starting when children are very young, parents help interpret the world to their children and help their children regulate their moods and emotional reactions. They communicate to a child that he or she is loved and valued, and contribute to the child's developing self-esteem. Parents teach and socialize their children both directly through instruction and indirectly by the example they set in their own behavior and in their relationships with others. Parents also transmit and reinforce cultural values and religious beliefs.

Adults have higher expectations of their school-age children and increasingly hold them accountable for their behavior. Yet parents spend about half as much time with children five to twelve years old as they do with children under five years. As their children become older, parents tend to use more discussion and reasoning with their children and expect greater compliance with their instructions. However, parents differ markedly in their parenting skills and parenting styles.

Baumrind described three major parenting styles: authoritarian, permissive, and authoritative. Parents may use all of these styles to different degrees at different times, but commonly one predominant style characterizes their behavior.

Authoritarian parents value obedience, respect for authority, conformity, work, tradition, and the preservation of order. They attempt to shape and control the behaviors and attitudes of their children, and expect them to accept the word of their parents on what is right and wrong. Authoritarian parents do not value independence and individuality. Typically, they tend to be demanding of their children and not very responsive to their needs. Boys raised in these families tend to be hostile and have low self-esteem; the girls are somewhat dependent, lacking in ambition, and unlikely to exhibit high levels of school achievement.

Permissive parents have a tolerant and accepting attitude toward their children's impulses, including sexual and aggressive impulses. They make few demands for mature behavior and prefer to allow their children to make their own decisions and regulate their own behavior. These parents tend to avoid using punishment, and wherever possible also avoid asserting their authority and imposing control on their children. Interestingly, children raised in these families tend to have characteristics very similar to those of children from authoritarian families.

Authoritative parents, by contrast, have clear expectations for mature behavior and set very clear standards for their children. They tend to enforce rules and standards but at the same time encourage independence and individuality. These parents value open communication with their children, consider their child's viewpoint, and encourage verbal give and take. Children raised in these families tend to be responsible and independent, showing social competence and maturity at all ages.

Other Factors Affecting Social Development

A multitude of factors influence children's social skills and competence. We discuss here a few of the most important of these factors.

Family Factors. Family environment has been shown to have a major influence on the child's social development. Economic and social changes in recent years have led to an enormous increase in the number of families in which both parents work, often out of necessity, to meet the financial needs of the family. Research has shown that families benefit from the increased financial resources and the satisfaction that both parents derive from their work. However, there is a price to pay in terms of the decreased availability of parents to children and the decreased sharing of leisure activities and social opportunities. In addition, although fathers are increasingly likely to share domestic and child-rearing responsibilities, the burden of child care still most likely falls on the mother, despite the fact that she is working.

School-age children often report feelings of dissatisfaction due to not having sufficient time with their parents; a complaint often echoed by their mothers. Nonetheless, school-age children appear to be more able to understand the reasons why both their parents must work and to tolerate more time alone than can preschool-age children. There is evidence to suggest that girls, in particular, benefit from the role models provided by their working mothers and that they tend to attain higher academic grades and professional achievement than girls whose mothers do not work outside of the home. In working-class families, this finding may not be true for boys, as their mothers often work out of necessity due to their fathers' low-paying jobs. Some studies have shown that the relationship between fathers and sons may be undermined in these families, with the sons having problems with both academic performance and social development.

As a consequence of the growing number of families in which both parents work, an increasing number of children return to empty homes where they are not supervised after school—the so-called *latchkey* children. These children often have to contend with feelings of loneliness and isolation, and those who live in inner-city, high-crime neighborhoods are more at risk of exposure to dangerous incidents. Children also may be at risk of accidents in the home due to the lack of supervision. Research has suggested that as latchkey children enter adolescence, they are more likely to abuse drugs and alcohol.

Poverty. Children in single parent families—whether as the result of birth to a single mother, divorce, parental death, or out-of-state employment—are at particular risk, because many of these families are headed by mothers with few financial resources. By far the largest proportion of families living in poverty are those headed by single mothers; this increasing phenomenon has been termed *the feminization of poverty.* Changes in the economy and reductions in government programs that provide assistance to the poor also play a large role in the growth of poverty.

Children reared in poverty are at risk for behavioral and emotional disturbances and school failure. These children suffer from compromised parenting, exposure to the disorganization and lawlessness of very poor neighborhoods, and limited opportunities to develop skills and build self-esteem.

Clinical Problems Involving Peer and Parent Relationships

A variety of problem behaviors manifest themselves in a child's social relationships and may result from the child's failure to negotiate the age-appropriate developmental tasks.

Disruptive Behavioral Disorders.   Although clinicians describe Oppositional Defiant Disorder and Conduct Disorder as primarily adolescent phenomena, these disorders often appear during the school-age years. Paradoxically, argumentative children who openly defy their parents are frequently asking for the parents to assert a greater degree of control. Clinicians may need to engage the parents of these children in psychotherapy to help them understand the issues that prevent them from taking effective control of their children.

Children with Conduct Disorder engage in frankly antisocial behavior, including getting into fights, committing petty crime, and inflicting deliberate cruelty on peers and animals. They exhibit an alarming lack of concern for the feelings of others, which signals deficits in the development of a conscience. It is important in these cases to consider the social and familial factors that have interfered with the child's moral development. In many cases such children have been victims of abusive or neglectful treatment, and their parents have failed to set limits on their behavior, provide appropriate role models, and instruct them on appropriate social conventions.

The Socially Inhibited Child. The child who is socially inhibited, anxious, or shy lies at the other end of the behavioral spectrum. Such children are less often referred for treatment but are at no less risk in terms of problems in social relationships. There is some evidence that the child's temperament is an important contributor, because the child who tends to avoid novel stimuli and hangs back in social situations—the so-called *slow-to-warm-up child*—is much more likely to have difficulties in new social situations. But it is also important to look at family and environmental factors that may be failing to promote assertiveness and self-confidence in these children. Frequently, these children have problems with depression and anxiety as well as significant problems with their self-image and self-esteem.

THE DEVELOPMENT OF SELF-ESTEEM

A common theme of this chapter has been the importance of self-esteem in the school-age child. School-age children start to evaluate themselves in relation to task demands, their peers, and their aspirations. High self-esteem during childhood predicts satisfaction in later life, whereas low self-esteem predicts depression, anxiety, poor school performance, and problematic social relationships.

Self-esteem develops gradually during the school-age years and depends to a large degree on success in the academic and social tasks of childhood. Children tend to judge themselves as they are reflected in the appraisal of significant others, particularly parents, teachers, and peers. Thus, children who are accepted feel good about themselves; those constantly criticized or rejected view themselves as inadequate.

Erik Erikson, a psychoanalyst, drew attention to the importance of feelings of competence and mastery as critical to the development of self-esteem. Erikson described a series of developmental tasks that take on particular relevance at different stages of development. If a child fails to resolve the major issue of a given stage, he or she will encounter difficulties in negotiating subsequent stages. In the school-age child, Erikson described the key developmental issue as involving *industry* (a sense of effectiveness, mastery, and competence) *versus inferiority.* He believed that children at this age derive confidence and a sense of self-worth from mastery and achievement in many different domains.

One of the most important factors in developing self-esteem is the nature of the child's relationship with his or her parents. Parents who enjoy their child, are responsive to his or her needs, provide consistent emotional support, and are involved and interested in their child's achievements are likely to promote the development of their child's self-esteem. However, it is important that parents' expectations be realistic and not overly ambitious, to avoid the child's experiencing feelings of failure at disappointing his or her parents. Children also benefit from having clear and consistent rules and expectations from their parents (as described in the section on parenting styles).

Other important influences on self-esteem include teachers, siblings, and peers, as well as community institutions. Minority children may be at special risk if the culture does not value the attributes of their particular ethnic group. Immigrant children and children from lower socioeconomic classes face a special challenge as they attempt to acculturate while at the same time trying to maintain a sense of their unique cultural identity.

Having reviewed some of the major developmental accomplishments of middle childhood and some of the clinical problems that may arise when development does not proceed smoothly, we now turn to important general principles of assessment and treatment for the school-age child.

PRINCIPLES OF ASSESSMENT AND TREATMENT

Conducting a thorough and rigorous assessment of the school-age child is essential before undertaking treatment. This complex task requires the ability to synthesize information regarding the child's past and current behavior from multiple sources, such as parents, other family members, teachers, school psychologists, and camp leaders. In fact, information can be obtained from anyone who has the opportunity to interact with the child on a regular basis. Past medical and psychiatric records and details of academic or psychological testing can also provide valuable information.

Assessment

Assessment takes place in several phases. The first step should be a separate meeting with the parents, so they can speak freely about their concerns. This information is an essential part of the diagnostic assessment. The next step is to assess the child directly.

Parent Interview. The parent interview serves many different functions. One of the first goals of the parent interview is to help set the family at ease and to gain the parents' support for the evaluation. By the time a child is referred for psychiatric assessment, there has generally been a fairly lengthy history of troublesome symptoms. Parents often experience anger, frustration, and feelings of failure for being unable to resolve these problems without the help of a mental health professional. Parents may need support in dealing with these issues.

The parent interview also provides an opportunity both to assess the family's need and motivation for treatment. Frequently, one parent blames the other for the presenting pathology, and the symptoms of the child may highlight important disagreements between the parents on matters of discipline and child rearing practices. It is often helpful to focus on the strengths of the family and child, while at the same time giving an honest and informed opinion of the issues involved and potential treatment strategies.

The parent interview provides information about the impact of the child's problems on the family. It may lead to the decision to meet individually with one parent or with smaller subgroups of the family, especially when there is reason to suspect abuse or extramarital affairs. Finally, the parent interview is often used to advise parents how to prepare the child for the first meeting with the therapist.

Child Interview. The diagnostic interview helps set the stage for establishing an effective therapeutic alliance with the child. It is important to communicate to the child that his or her problems are important and being taken seriously. Paramount is an ability to take a flexible approach and to establish ways to place the child at ease in what is often a new and somewhat threatening situation.

Important information about the child can be derived from the child's appearance and behavior (based even on observations made in the waiting room), such as the child's level of activity and the child's response to being separated from the parent. Early in the session, it is customary to investigate the child's understanding of the purpose of the consultation and to clarify the limits of confidentiality.

In working with school-age children, a variety of techniques may be used, including play, to put the child at ease. Often in this age group, children will not speak directly about their concerns, but information about feelings and family dynamics may emerge in the context of play. Frequently, the play therapy session will provide important diagnostic information. The therapist should pay attention to the spontaneity and quality of the child's play. It is important to notice how the child engages the therapist, as well as the child's degree of reciprocity. Recurrent themes or interuptions in play may indicate important conflicts or areas of concern for the child. Play can also provide information about the child's level of cognitive and social development. Table 1.1 lists the major areas of inquiry to cover during the assessment of both the family and the child.

The Importance of the Family in Treatment

In treating school-age children it is often important to treat the family. As highlighted in earlier sections, the family has a major influence on all aspects of the child's development and adjustment. Family conflicts are frequently associated with psychiatric pathology in the child, and, conversely, the child's symptoms may lead to stress on the parents and other siblings. Thus, it is important to attempt to assess the coalitions between family members, the lines of authority, and the presence or absence of appropriate boundaries between children and parents.

Family Systems. The principles of "family systems" underlie all models of family therapy and may be summarized as follows. First, people in families are closely connected, and it is helpful to look at the nature of these connections rather than just focusing on individual members. Second, family members who interact repeatedly over time establish predictable patterns of behavior that may be influenced by historical, personal, or cultural influences. Psychiatric difficulties arise when these patterns of family interaction inhibit or prevent individual development, or interfere with the attempts of the family to devise solutions to the inevitable problems that arise. Third, families frequently resist and subtly undermine interventions aimed at changing existing patterns of functioning. Frequently, the presenting "problem child" masks other problems in the family, such as

Table 1.1
Assessment of the School-Age Child

Identifying data

History of presenting problem (as defined by both the parents and the child)

Past psychiatric history

Developmental history

- Pregnancy: maternal nutritional status, exposure to drugs and alcohol
- Birth history
- Developmental milestones
- Attachment history: significant separation experiences
- Neglect, physical and sexual abuse
- Peer and sibling relationships
- School history; academic problems

Substance abuse history

Past medical history

Current medications

Family history

- Psychiatric problems and treatment
- Substance abuse history in family members
- Significant medical problems in family members

Mental status examination

- General observations: grooming, tics or motor movements, nutrition, signs of abuse, sociability
- Kinetics: psychomotor retardation or agitation
- Language: maturity and vocabulary, intelligibility, rate of speech
- Affect: range and quality of mood; symptoms of depression, mania, or anxiety; neurovegetative symptoms
- Thought process: loosening of associations, logicality, formal thought disorder
- Thought content: delusions, ideas of reference, paranoia, obsessions, compulsions
- Perceptions: illusions, hallucinations
- Cognition: orientation, attention span, cognitive ability, memory, insight
- Capacity for symbolic and imaginative play: dreams, fantasies

marital problems. Only after the marital problems (or other underlying family problems) are dealt with is the child likely to improve. This is illustrated in the following case.

WILLIAM

William, an eight-year-old boy, manifested oppositional behavior at school and at home. He was a spirited and engaging child who went out of his way to provoke his parents and teachers. His mother, Laura, appeared passive, overwhelmed, and unable to follow even simple recommendations regarding time-outs and behavior management. A closer examination of the family dynamics revealed that Laura was depressed and angry at her husband, who worked long hours and took little initiative when it came to controlling William's behavior. For Laura, William's oppositionality was a way to expose her husband's absence from the family and his lack of involvement as both a father and husband. It was not until the difficulties in the parent's marriage were addressed that both parents were able to unite and enforce a simple and effective behavior modification program that led to a rapid resolution of William's problems.

Play Therapy

The use of play is one of the fundamental differences between treating school-age children and working with adults. Children generally are unable to sit for long periods and talk about their problems, as we expect of adults. What they will do, however, is engage spontaneously through the medium of play. Melanie Klein, one of the founders of child psychoanalysis, was one of the first clinicians to promote the use of play as a therapeutic technique with children. In fact, she believed that it was possible to gain a direct view of the child's unconscious fantasies and conflicts by observing their play. The following case illustrates how play therapy can reveal issues that children cannot or will not articulate during an interview.

MARTHA

Martha, a seven-year-old girl, was referred to therapy after developing severe constipation, which did not respond to normal medical interventions. In play therapy, Martha was silent and unwilling to answer questions but quickly showed an interest in playing with dolls in the therapist's office. Although the dolls' clothes were glued firmly to the bodies, Martha became fixated on trying to undress them. In subsequent play, themes of sexual abuse emerged. Inquiry of her parents revealed that Martha's unemployed uncle had recently moved into the family's apartment. When the therapist questioned Martha about her uncle, she reported that her uncle had been sexually abusing her and that she was too frightened to tell anyone because of his threats to retaliate.

A major task in working with the school-age child is to put into words the material emerging in play and in this way help the child acknowledge his or her feelings. Interruptions in play generally signal anxiety, and paying close attention to the timing of play disruptions often helps reveal the underlying significance of the child's symptoms. The following case illustrates this point.

EMILY

Emily, a seven-year-old girl, was referred to a therapist after several episodes of bed-wetting and nightmares. In play therapy with dolls, she created elaborate family scenes enacting daily routines. The therapist noticed that Emily would rush out for a "bathroom break" at the point in the story when the father was getting into the car to go to work. Exploration of this theme revealed that Emily worried that her father would not return home from work. Although there had been no change in her home situation, Emily told the therapist that her best friend's father had been hospitalized for a malignant brain tumor, which had presented with severe headaches. Emily was terrified of the same thing happening to her own father, who had a history of migraine headaches. With some simple clarification of the difference between brain cancer and her father's migraine, Emily's symptoms rapidly resolved. We can see that the play interruption in this case was not a random event but contained useful information about the causes of Emily's anxiety.

Child's Symptoms as a Reflection of Underlying Problems in the Parent

As we would expect, parents frequently bring their children into treatment, but in many cases, such as Peter's in the next example, it turns out that the child's problem expresses a conflict that resides with one of the parents.

PETER

Peter, a ten-year-old boy with Oppositional Defiant Disorder, was referred with his family for treatment. His oppositionality appeared to be a problem mainly for his single mother, Anne. Clinical explorations revealed that Anne had been raised in a family with an authoritarian and tyrannical father. Her response to this environment was to avoid direct conflict, and she carried this response over to her own parenting, exhibiting an overly permissive style. For Anne, trying to set limits on Peter's behavior brought back traumatic memories of her father's harsh control of the family.

The process by which parents' symptoms transfer to their children is complex. In some cases, the parent fails to provide support for aspects of the child's development due to the very absence of these qualities in the parent, as in the case just described. In other situations, the child learns in subtle ways to model him- or herself on the behavior of the parent. Further, it is likely that biological or temperamental variables may predispose the child to certain symptoms.

These issues should be kept in mind when assessing the child. They not only shed light on the child's symptoms but may indicate a need to involve parents in their own treatment to address the issues that are affecting their parenting.

Countertransference

The term *countertransference* describes those feelings experienced by the *clinician* in relation to the patient—strong emotional reactions toward the patient that are triggered by the earlier experiences of the therapist. Unresolved issues of the therapist may interfere with the ability to work effectively and objectively with the patient.

Working closely with a child may bring up powerful emotions. It is common for therapists to experience feelings of anger toward parents whom they may perceive as neglectful or unsupportive of their child. This is particularly true if the therapist has experienced similar issues with his or her own parents, and it is easy to get caught up in a situation of blaming the parents of the child in treatment and to lose the objectivity necessary to be helpful to the family.

A common phenomenon of working with children is for the treatment to call up feelings and memories from the therapist's own childhood, especially those associated with issues that were particularly problematic when the therapist was the same age as the child he or she is treating. These conflicts can lead to difficulties and may interfere with treatment, especially in cases where the therapist's issues were not fully resolved. The following case illustrates this point.

SHEILA

Sheila, a thirty-three-year-old psychiatry trainee working with a challenging and underprivileged inner-city population, experienced more than usual difficulties interacting with the families assigned to her. She was quick to judge and criticize the families and lacked empathy with their situations. What emerged in supervision was that Sheila's family had been dysfunctional: her father had been unusually abusive and critical, and her mother had been unable to protect her from his assaults. As a therapist, Sheila saw her role as providing protection for her child patients from abusive family situations. Although in many of her cases there were elements of maltreatment, her zeal in blaming the parents clearly reverberated with her own personal experiences and prevented her from being able to establish a therapeutic and helpful relationship with the families who had come to the clinic seeking help.

Managed Care Issues

Providing treatment for children and families in today's health care system demands an ability to work within the limits imposed by managed care. Insurance benefits for individual and family psychotherapy are frequently limited to a restricted number of sessions per year, and inpatient benefits may have a lifetime maximum. This raises challenges in situations where we may believe that longer-term treatment is necessary to address severe psychiatric disorders, and in many of these cases it may be up to the family to pay for treatment out of pocket. In addition, when insurance is available, many insurance companies have a list of providers who are authorized to provide treatment.

Our role is often to help the families negotiate these issues and to help them become effective advocates for their children. Educating families about the different treatment options and helping families make the most of their benefits are becoming increasingly important tasks for the therapist.

Treating school-age children can be one of the most rewarding experiences in the mental health professions. Children in this age group are often very receptive to treatment suggestions and take pleasure in mastering new information. In addition, the maturational and developmental changes these children are undergoing will often work synergistically with the therapist to support the therapeutic work. Paying close attention to the child's developmental issues, involving the family in treatment, and providing the child with the opportunity to be heard and understood in a respectful and empathic manner are the keys to success in treatment.

NOTES

P. 2, *Between the ages of five and seven years, and following a maturational timetable:* Cole, M., & Cole, S. R. (1993). *The development of children* (2nd ed.). New York: Scientific American Books, pp. 441–444.

P. 3, *Children in this age group . . . to remember things:* Zigler, E. F., & Stevenson, M. F. (1993). *Children in a changing world: Development and social issues* (2nd ed.). Pacific Grove, CA: Brooks/Cole, pp. 413–415.

P. 4, *Piaget termed this new level of thinking:* Zigler, E. F., & Stevenson, M. F. (1993). *ibid.*, pp. 415–425.

P. 6, *the developmental sequence of middle childhood is similar across all cultures:* Cole, M., & Cole, S. R. (1993). *ibid.*, p. 461.

P. 7, *Jerome Kagan noted that children:* Zigler, E. F., & Stevenson, M. F. (1993). *ibid.*, p. 436.

P. 7, *Children whose parents take an active interest . . . have high levels of academic achievement:* Cole, M., & Cole, S. R. (1993). *ibid.*, p. 505.

P. 8, *Schools that demonstrate a strong commitment:* Jencks, C. (1972). *Inequality: A reassessment of the effect of family and schooling in America.* New York: Basic Books.

P. 9, *Attention Deficit Hyperactivity Disorder:* American Psychiatric Association. (1994). *Diagnostic and statistical manual of mental disorders* (4th ed.). Washington, DC: Author.

P. 9, *One school of thought claims:* Hechtman, L. (1991). Developmental, neurobiological, and psychosocial aspects of hyperactivity, impulsivity and inattention. In M. Lewis (Ed.), *Child and adolescent psychiatry: A comprehensive textbook.* Baltimore: Williams & Wilkins, p. 318.

P. 9, *Others argue that the symptoms:* Chess, S., & Thomas, A. (1986). *Temperament in clinical practice.* New York: Guilford, pp. 233–236.

P. 10, *Genetic factors, toxic events . . . have been implicated:* Apin, I. (1988). Disorders of higher cerebral function in preschool children. *American Journal of the Disabled Child, 142,* 1119–1124.

P. 10, *Boys appear to engage in more:* Cole, M., & Cole, S. R. (1993). *ibid.,* pp. 538–539.

P. 11, *Competitive sports organized by adults:* Cole, M., & Cole, S. R. (1993). *ibid.,* pp. 520–521.

P. 11, *Psychoanalytic theories suggest:* Gemelli, R. (1996). *Normal child and adolescent development.* Washington, DC: American Psychiatric Press, pp. 366–369.

P. 12, *Lawrence Kohlberg suggested a theory:* Zigler, E. F., & Stevenson, M. F. (1993). *ibid.,* pp. 456–462.

P. 12, *When entering a new peer group:* Puttallaz, M., & Gottman, J. M. (1981). Social skills and group acceptance. In S. R. Asher & J. M. Gottman (Eds.), *The development of children's friendships.* Cambridge, England: Cambridge University Press.

P. 12, *Aggressive children paradoxically tend:* Dodge, K. A., Pettit, G. S., McClaskey, C. L., & Brown, M. M. (1986). Social competence in children. *Monographs of the Society for Research in Child Development. 51*(2, Serial No. 213).

P. 12, *A coercive family atmosphere will:* Dishion, T. J. (1990). The family ecology of boys' peer relations in middle childhood. *Child Development, 61,* 874–892.

P. 13, *Significantly, peer rejection tends:* Parker, J. G., & Asher, S. R. (1987). Peer relations and later personal adjustment: Are low-accepted children "at risk"? *Psychological Bulletin, 102,* 357–389.

P. 13, *Yet parents spend about half as much time with children five to twelve years old:* Hill, C. R., & Stafford, F. P. (1980). Parental care of children: Time diary estimates of quantity, predictability and variety. *Journal of Human Resources, 15,* 219–239.

P. 13, *Baumrind described three major parenting styles:* Baumrind, D. (1971). Current patterns of parental authority. *Developmental Psychology Monographs, 4* (1, Part 2).

P. 15, *School-age children often report feelings of dissatisfaction:* Zigler, E. F., & Stevenson, M. F. (1993). *ibid.,* p. 479.

P. 15, *an increasing number of children return to empty homes . . . the so-called latchkey children:* Zigler, E. F., & Stevenson, M. F. (1993). *ibid.,* p. 480–481.

P. 17, *the child who tends to avoid novel stimuli and hangs back:* Chess, S., & Thomas, A. (1986). *ibid.,* pp. 34–36.

P. 18, *Erik Erikson, a psychoanalyst:* Erikson, E. H. (1963). *Childhood and society* (2nd ed.). New York: Norton.

P. 21, *The principles of "family systems":* Barnes, G. G. (1994). Family therapy. In M. Rutter, E. Taylor, & L. Hersov (Eds.), *Child and adolescent psychiatry: Modern approaches* (3rd ed.). Oxford, England: Blackwell, p. 946.

P. 23, *Melanie Klein, one of the founders:* Klein, M. (1975). *The psycho-analysis of children.* New York: Free Press, pp. 16–34.

FOR FURTHER READING

Cole, M., & Cole, S. R. (1993). Cognitive and biological attainments of middle childhood. In Cole, M., & Cole, S. R. (Eds.), *The development of children* (2nd ed., pp. 437–467). New York: Scientific American Books.

Cole, M., & Cole, S. R. (1993). Schooling and development in middle childhood. In Cole, M., & Cole, S. R. (Eds.), *The development of children* (2nd ed., pp. 469–513). New York: Scientific American Books.

Cole, M., & Cole, S. R. (1993). The social relations of middle childhood. In Cole, M., & Cole, S. R. (Eds.), *The development of children* (2nd ed., pp. 515–562). New York: Scientific American Books.

Cox, A. D. (1994). Diagnostic appraisal. In M. Rutter, E. Taylor, & L. Hersov (Eds.), *Child and adolescent psychiatry: Modern approaches* (3rd ed., pp. 22–33). Oxford, England: Blackwell.

Kaplan, H. I., Sadock, B. J., & Grebb, J. A. (1994). Theories of personality and psychopathology: Sigmund Freud: Founder of classic psychoanalysis.

In H. I. Kaplan & B. J. Sadock (Eds.), *Synopsis of psychiatry: Behavioral sciences, clinical psychiatry* (7th ed., pp. 245–247). Baltimore: Williams and Wilkins.

Kaplan, H. I., Sadock, B. J., & Grebb, J. A. (1994). Theories of personality and psychopathology: Erik Erikson. In H. I. Kaplan & B. J. Sadock (Eds.), *Synopsis of psychiatry: Behavioral sciences, clinical psychiatry* (7th ed., pp. 260–264). Baltimore: Williams and Wilkins.

Kaplan, H. I., Sadock, B. J., & Grebb, J. A. (1994). Contributions of the psychosocial sciences to human behavior: Jean Piaget. In H. I. Kaplan & B. J. Sadock (Eds.), *Synopsis of psychiatry: Behavioral sciences, clinical psychiatry* (7th ed., pp. 157–161). Baltimore: Williams and Wilkins.

Lewis, M. (1991). Normal growth and development. In J. M. Wiener (Ed.), *Textbook of child and adolescent psychiatry* (pp. 25–39). Washington, DC: American Psychiatric Press.

Malone, C. A. (1991). Family therapy. In J. M. Wiener (Ed.), *Textbook of child and adolescent psychiatry* (pp. 605–616). Washington, DC: American Psychiatric Press.

Rutter, M., & Rutter, M. (1993). The growth of social relationships. In *Developing minds: Challenge and continuity across the life span* (pp. 110–155). New York: Basic Books.

Zigler, E. F., & Stevenson, M. F. (1993). Physical development during middle childhood. In E. F. Zigler & M. F. Stevenson (Eds.), *Children in a changing world: Development and social issues* (2nd ed., pp. 386–409). Pacific Grove, CA: Brooks/Cole.

Zigler, E. F., & Stevenson, M. F. (1993). Cognitive development during middle childhood. In E. F. Zigler & M. F. Stevenson (Eds.), *Children in a changing world: Development and social issues* (2nd ed., pp. 410–449). Pacific Grove, CA: Brooks/Cole.

Zigler, E. F., & Stevenson, M. F. (1993). Social and emotional development during middle childhood. In E. F. Zigler & M. F. Stevenson (Eds.), *Children in a changing world: Development and social issues* (2nd ed., pp. 450–487). Pacific Grove, CA: Brooks/Cole.

2

OBSESSIVE-COMPULSIVE DISORDER, PHOBIAS, AND TRAUMA

Sharon E. Williams, Julie A. Collier, and Zakee Matthews

Therapist: Why don't you like to go to school?
Bobby: Because I don't.
Therapist: What happens when you go to school? How do you feel?
Bobby: Scared. I feel worried when my mom is ready to leave.
Therapist: Why do you feel scared and worried when your mom leaves?
Bobby: I don't want her to go. I sometimes worry that something will happen to her. Then I start to get upset.
Therapist: What happens when you get upset?
Bobby: Sometimes I cry. Then I tell the teacher that I need to call my mom to come and get me.

The start of school is both an exciting and intimidating time for children. As children begin their formal education, the focus of their environment shifts from home to school. The expected changes and transitions of the early school years carry with them some degree of anxiety, which is a normal part of development. Such issues as making and losing friends, learning new subjects, changing schools, and experiencing changes in the family structure with divorce or the addition of new siblings are just a few of the instances that can create anxiety and disappointment.

Although brief situational anxiety of brief duration is common in most children, some children experience a level of anxiety that impairs their social and academic functioning and disrupts normal development. Studies have found that as many as 17 percent of children have anxiety disorders. These significant numbers substantiate the importance of these disorders in children.

In this chapter we explore the issue of anxiety in children, looking specifically at the diagnoses that are associated with this age group. We review the assessment process and discuss the symptoms associated with Obsessive-Compulsive Disorder, Separation Anxiety Disorder, phobias, and Posttraumatic Stress Disorder. We also discuss Panic Disorder and Generalized Anxiety Disorder, although these conditions are not as prevalent in this age group. Finally, we review treatment techniques.

ASSESSMENT

Effective treatment is only possible when it follows a thorough assessment and accurate diagnosis of the problem. As the clinician, you must determine whether anxiety represents a transient reaction to a recent stressor or developmental phase, or is a manifestation of a more serious disorder. You must also identify the extent to which the symptoms are interfering with the child's current level of functioning.

The process of assessing a child with anxiety symptoms does not differ greatly from the assessment process of any other disorder or problem, and must include a thorough developmental, behavioral, medical, academic, and family history. Highlighted in the following section are some of the areas of particular relevance to the assessment of anxiety symptoms in children.

Medical History

It is very important to obtain a thorough medical history, including family medical history, during the initial assessment. A number of medical disorders are associated with anxiety symptoms.

Endocrine disorders such as hyperthyroidism or hypoglycemia, for example, can present with anxiety as the primary symptom. This was the case for one nine-year-old boy who complained that he could sometimes feel his heart racing. This symptom could have been interpreted as a primary anxiety problem, but was actually a symptom of hyperthyroidism. Additionally, medications (for example, steroids or beta agonists) prescribed for medical illnesses can induce or exacerbate feelings of anxiety in children. It is important to determine when the child last had a physical exam and to ascertain an accurate list of medications the child is currently taking. Every child who presents with anxiety need not be immediately referred to her pediatrician. However, if there are any new medical complaints associated with the onset of anxiety, or if there is a family history of medical problems that are commonly associated with anxiety symptoms, a complete medical evaluation is warranted. Concerns about the impact of prescription medications on anxiety symptoms should be referred to the prescribing physician. A change of medication or alteration of dosage may alleviate the symptoms.

Family History

It is essential that you obtain a thorough family assessment that includes a family history of mood and anxiety disorders as well as the parents' typical responses to displays of anxiety or fear by the child. There is strong evidence suggesting that anxiety disorders may have a genetic component. However, it can be difficult to differentiate the contribution of genetics from the impact of growing up in a family with anxious relatives who model fearful behavior.

When a child presents with an anxiety disorder, the family has often already tried several techniques to deal with the problem. These solutions can range from the parent's lying in bed for several hours with a child who is fearful of the dark and will not go to sleep, to warfare in the family as both the child and parent refuse to give in to the other's request. The end result is a disruption of the family system that can often lead to tension, anger, and frustration among family members, including siblings. You should interview the child and the parents as to the ways in which the family has changed since the appearance of the anxiety. Routines, roles, and dynamics should all be explored—including the period before the anxiety-related behavior started, once it ensued, and the current state of affairs.

You should also investigate the parenting strategies of both parents to assess whether or not they are in agreement about the nature and etiology of the anxiety, as well as about the ways in which to deal with it. Parents will often have differing opinions as to why the behavior is present—for example, they may characterize the child as troubled, emotional, or manipulative—and how the behavior should be handled (give him time, it's a phase, snap out of it, just do it). Even under the best of circumstances, tension can arise between parents when their relationship is significantly affected for a prolonged time (whether caused by disagreements about how to handle the child's behavior or by increased time spent apart dealing with the child). Similarly, siblings can also be affected. For example, their routine and activities may be disrupted by not being able to go out because a brother or sister is scared of crowded places or afraid to be without one particular parent.

Other stressors that may bear on a child's complaints of anxiety include increased family discord, such as marital conflict, separations, and divorce, and any other recent losses or perceived threats of loss. You should also inquire about exposure to recent frightening or upsetting events. For example, one child with whom we worked had witnessed gang-related violence in his neighborhood, which led to the onset of anxious, fearful behavior. In another case, a child's school anxiety was related to a stern reprimand from a teacher. Other traumatic events, such as physical and sexual abuse, can also lead to significant anxiety.

School History

Along with an assessment of the family, contact with the child's school teachers can prove to be very beneficial. Does the child exhibit anxious behavior at school? Are there additional behavioral difficulties that interfere with the child's academic performance or peer relationships? Occasionally we hear from a teacher that he believes a particular child has "ADHD." Upon closer examination, however, we find that the fidgety behavior and difficulty with concentration are related to anxiety rather than to attention problems or hyperactivity. Please note, however, that anxious children do not always exhibit negative, problematic behavior in school. In some cases, a child may become extremely focused on his schoolwork and perform quite well. For example, nine-year-old Joseph, who was doing well in school, came to our clinic because of irritability and difficulties with sleep. Upon investigation, it was revealed that Joseph worried a great deal about his school performance due to an overwhelming fear of his parents' disappointment if he were to do poorly in school.

If the anxious behavior occurs primarily at school, you should be alert for the possibility of a learning disability or a difficult peer situation. Anxious behavior that predominates at home rather than at school is often indicative of a family-based problem. This was the case for an eight-year-old girl who was identified by her mother as "always worried." Bedtime was particularly difficult because of her fear of the dark. Our assessment revealed that the child performed well at school, and, according to the teacher, she did not appear unduly anxious or worried. Our assessment further revealed that the child's father had a drinking problem that led to many arguments between the parents at night. Her symptoms waxed and waned depending on the severity of the father's drinking and the level of conflict in the family.

Assessment Measures

There are a number of assessment instruments available for measuring anxiety in children. These measures can help you differentiate pathological anxiety from the fears and concerns that are part of normal development. (See Table 2.1 for some of the most commonly used anxiety assessment tools.)

Table 2.1
Assessment Tools

Semistructured Interviews

Schedule for Affective Disorders and Schizophrenia in School-Aged Children (K-SADS; Puig-Antich & Chambers, 1978)

Anxiety Disorders Interview Schedule for Children (ADIS-C; Silverman & Nelles, 1988)

Children's Anxiety Evaluation Form (CAEF; Hoegn-Saric, Maisami, & Weigand, 1987)

Child Assessment Schedule (CAS; Hodges & Fitch, 1979)

Child and Adolescent Psychiatric Assessment (CAPA; Angld, Pendergast, Cox, et al., in press)

Yale-Brown Obsessive Compulsive Scale (YBOCS; Goodman, Price, Rasmussen, et al., 1989)

Structured Interviews

Diagnostic Interview for Children and Adolescents (DICA; Welner et al., 1987)

Diagnostic Interview Schedule for Children (DISC; Costello, Edelbrock, & Dulcan, 1985)

NIMH Diagnostic Interview Schedule for Children (Shaffer et al., 1996)

Cognitive and educational testing may also be warranted when there is school-related anxiety that may be due to an underlying learning disability. Projective tests, such as the Rorschach, Thematic Apperception Test, or the Children's Apperception Test, may also be helpful in clarifying diagnostically complex cases.

Cultural Issues

As when making any diagnosis, you need to consider cultural values and issues when working with minority populations. In many racial or ethnic groups, receiving help from mental health professionals is taboo. Instead, problems are dealt with in the

Table 2.1   *(continued)*

Parent-Teacher Ratings

Child Behavior Checklist (CBCL; Achenback & Edelbrock, 1983)

Personality Inventory for Children (PIC; Wirt et al., 1977)

Self-Report Measures

Revised Chldren's Manifest Anxiety Scale (RCMAS; Reynolds & Richmond, 1978)

State-Trait Anxiety Inventory for Children (STAIC; Spielberger, Edwards, & Lushene, 1973)

Fear Survey Schedule for Children-Revised (FSSC-R; Ollendick, 1983)

Social Anxiety Scale for Children (SASC; La Greca, Dandes, Wick, et al., 1988)

Multidimensional Anxiety Scale for Children (MASC; March, Stallings, Parker, et al., 1994)

Social Phobia Anxiety Inventory for Children (SPAI-C; Turner, Beidel, Dancu, et al., 1989)

Visual Analogue Scale for Anxiety-Revised (Bernstein & Garfinkel, 1992)

Source: Adapted from Bernstein, G. A., Borchardt, C. M., & Perwein, A. R. (1996). Anxiety disorders in children and adolescents: A review of the past ten years. *Journal of the American Academy of Child and Adolescent Psychiatry, 35*(9), 1110–1119.

family or community. Anxiety can often be explained away as a phase or personality trait, or be ignored all together, making it less likely that the child and parents will seek treatment.

It is not uncommon for children in minority families to experience pressure from family members to perform well in school, particularly if they are first or second generation. This pressure may exist as a long-standing tradition in the culture or may be due to the parents' drive for the child to achieve in ways that the parents did not have the opportunity to achieve themselves. Many children see this pressure as commonplace and as an acceptable practice in their culture. In fact, many families will not present to a mental health clinician because the pressure, although at times difficult to manage, will appear to be the norm, as in the case that follows.

CHRISTINE

Christine was a seven-year-old first-generation Korean girl who was referred to us by her pediatrician when no physical etiology was found for numerous episodes of stomachaches and restless sleeping. Our evaluation revealed that her symptoms occurred prior to days when she would have a test in school, particularly in subjects on which she thought she would not get an A. Christine's fears about not doing well were related to a fear of disappointing her parents and extended family.

In working with families who present with these concerns, it is important to highlight the effect this pressure is having on the child while being respectful of the traditions and the drive to achieve that are mainstays within the culture.

Many children who come from high socioeconomic status (SES) families also can experience anxiety related to school performance or professional aspirations as a result of the success standards of their parents. Children as young as school age often report a drive to do well in order to achieve and go on to college and beyond.

SYMPTOMS AND DIAGNOSES

Anxiety can present in a number of different ways in children. In this next section we review the major areas of childhood anxiety disorders and their presentation. Some diagnoses are more common in children than are others, and some manifest differently in children than in adolescents or adults. We discuss these issues with respect to each disorder.

Obsessive-Compulsive Disorder

Children with Obsessive-Compulsive Disorder (OCD) experience obsessive thoughts, urges, and images that are anxiety provoking. In response to the obsessions, the children perform repetitive behaviors or engage in covert mental acts (such as counting) that serve to neutralize or alleviate their anxiety.

RYAN

Ryan, an African-American boy, was seven years old when his parents brought him to us for a psychological evaluation. For the previous two months he had been preoccupied with the possibility that he had "bad germs" on his hands. At first he would become anxious if his hands were visibly dirty. This concern progressed, however, to include the concern that his hands would be contaminated by germs if he touched any object that may have come in contact with something that was "dirty." In an attempt to alleviate overwhelming anxiety about germs and contamination, Ryan would wash his hands repeatedly.

The symptoms of childhood OCD are relatively consistent with those of adolescence and adulthood. Obsessions are usually seen in concert with compulsions; it is less common for obsessions or compulsions to present alone. Swedo, Rapoport, Leonard, and their colleagues at the National Institute of Mental Health (NIMH) identified the most common childhood compulsions as washing and cleaning, followed by checking, counting, repeating, touching, and straightening. The most common corresponding obsessions included fear of contamination and fear of harm to self or to a familiar person, followed by scrupulosity (excessive religiosity or scrutiny of one's thoughts or actions) and forbidden thoughts. Unlike most adolescents and adults, very young children may not recognize their obsessions as unusual.

In the NIMH sample described by Swedo, Rapoport, Leonard, and their colleagues, OCD symptoms can arise in children as young as seven years of age. They appear to be more common in boys, and many children with OCD have a family member with the disorder. The NIMH sample revealed numerous disorders that coexist with OCD, including tic disorders (30 percent of the sample had both OCD and tic disorder), Major Depression (26 percent), specific developmental disability (24 percent), simple phobias (17 percent), Overanxious Disorder (16 percent), Adjustment Disorder with Depressed Mood (13 percent), Oppositional Disorder (11 percent), Attention Deficit Disorder (10 percent), Conduct Disorder (7 percent), and Separation Anxiety Disorder (7 percent). For many children, OCD is a chronic disorder, the symptoms of which wax and wane over time.

Separation Anxiety Disorder

BOBBY

Eight-year-old Bobby, who was introduced at the beginning of the chapter, was brought to us by his parents because of his reluctance (and sometimes flat refusal) to attend school. Some mornings he could be coaxed into staying at school initially, but he would frequently become distressed and ask to go to the office to call his mother. At times he sounded so distraught that his mother would come pick him up. But it was not just school that proved difficult for Bobby. Most separations from his mother resulted in overt distress and tearfulness. Bobby stated that when he was not with his mother, he worried that something would happen to her and that she might never come back. His mother complained that at home Bobby frequently followed her around the house. Separations from his father were often difficult, but not to the degree that they were from his mother. Nighttime fears were also an issue, leading to difficulty falling asleep and frequent requests to join his parents in bed in the middle of the night.

Bobby exhibited many of the symptoms of Separation Anxiety Disorder (SAD). Additional symptoms that may be present include persistent and excessive worry that an untoward event (such as being kidnapped or getting lost) will lead to separation from a key attachment figure, repeated nightmares involving themes of separation, and recurrent complaints of physical symptoms (such as headaches, stomachaches, nausea, or vomiting) when separation from major attachment figures is anticipated.

SAD occurs most frequently in school-age children starting at about nine years of age and is more often found in girls than boys. The diagnosis can occur before the age of six years old, which qualifies it for a specifier of early onset in the *DSM-IV* nosology.

Phobias

Phobias encompass a wide variety of situations that produce anxiety in children. In this section, we examine Specific Phobia, Social Phobia, and school phobia.

A diagnosis of Specific Phobia (SP) is made when a child has a persistent fear of a specific object or situation. This fear leads to avoidance of the stimulus whenever possible, or to intense anxiety if the stimulus must be endured. Common phobic stimuli include animals, the dark, thunderstorms, medical procedures, escalators, or things that produce loud noises.

Many children experience fears during childhood that are considered to be part of normal development. A diagnosis of Specific Phobia, however, is warranted when the fear becomes disruptive to their daily activities, is accompanied by feelings of worry when the stimulus is encountered or believed to be encountered in the near future, and continues for a minimum of six months. Take, for example, the case of a Lori, a six-year-old African-American girl who expresses dislike for the dark and cannot sleep without a nightlight. Lori may protest a bit at bedtime, but with a nightlight she generally goes to sleep easily. Lori would be considered to have a normal childhood fear of the dark. If, on the other hand, she mounted vigorous protests at bedtime, could not be comforted with a nightlight, insisted on a parent being present for sleep to occur, or persistently avoided entering any dark room, we would make a diagnosis of Specific Phobia.

Children with Social Phobia (SOP) have a persistent fear of being embarrassed in social or performance situations. Debra Biedel identified a broad range of stressful social encounters reported in a sample of children with SOP. Eighty-eight percent of the children identified formal speaking as problematic, followed by eating in front of others (39.3 percent), going to parties (27.6 percent), writing in front of others (27.6 percent), using public restrooms (24.1 percent), speaking to authority figures (20.7 percent), and informal speaking (13 percent). To meet criteria for SOP, the child must demonstrate that he has the ability to engage in age-appropriate social activity, thereby ruling out the possibility that his behavior is due to immature social skills or a Pervasive Developmental Disorder.

When discussing SOP it is important to mention temperament and behavioral inhibition. Jerome Kagan and his colleagues at Harvard reported that 15 to 20 percent of Caucasian American children are temperamentally predisposed to be irritable as infants, shy and fearful as toddlers, and cautious, quiet, and introverted whey they reach school age. They estimate that approximately 30 percent of behaviorally inhibited children develop anxiety disorders, and that inhibited children who have a parent with an anxiety disorder are at highest risk for the development of an anxiety disorder over time.

Also related to both SOP and behavioral inhibition is the diagnosis of Selective Mutism. Although not classified in *DSM-IV* as an anxiety disorder, current conceptualizations of Selective Mutism relate it to shy, timid behavior or social anxiety. In the following passage, writer Jan Goben eloquently describes her experience as a child with Selective Mutism:

> I stopped talking when I started nursery school. It felt safer not to say anything.

I could talk to my dogs and cats. I'd sit for hours by the bird feeder, whistling and chirping and trying to make the birds understand me. I could talk to my brother, Greg, and my parents. But people outside my family were another story. If I talked to them, they might laugh. They might laugh like they laughed at Greg when he said he could see across the ocean to Japan.

Greg was bold and he didn't care. He knew he could see Japan, so it didn't matter what anyone said. But I didn't have his boldness. I knew just as many things as he did—I knew that God could see into our house from a painting in the hallway; I knew that I would someday marry Dr. Boyle, my pediatrician. I knew that elves lived in our chimney. But I also knew people would laugh at these facts, so I never told anyone.

As can be seen in this description, the refusal to talk in certain situations is generally not secondary to oppositional behavior but to shyness and anxiety about social interactions. Much more research on this disorder is needed so that we can understand the nature of the relationship between SOP, Selective Mutism, and the temperamental traits that may predispose a child to developing these disorders.

The occurrence of school phobia is largely related to Separation Anxiety Disorder and does not warrant a separate diagnosis in *DSM-IV.* Although it is true that some children resist going to school because of specific school-related problems, such as a class bully, a "mean" teacher, or a difficult subject, a greater percentage of children do not want to attend because of who or what they have to leave in order to go to school. There is another subgroup of children who resist going to school and meet criteria for SOP. This may be more common during the adolescent years, when peer relationships take on added significance, but school-age children who are shy or easily intimidated by social peer groups may resist school because of social situations.

Trauma-Related Anxiety

Children who have experienced a traumatic event often show symptoms of anxiety that fall under the classification of Post-traumatic Stress Disorder (PTSD) or Acute Stress Disorder (ASD). Under the *DSM-IV* classification of a traumatic event, the situation that induces psychological symptoms must produce in the person a perception of harm to herself or others and feelings of "fear, hopelessness, or horror." This definition allows for a wide range of experiences to be interpreted as traumatic. Situations that would not be considered significant to adults are often very disturbing to a child and can result in psychopathology. Anxiety in these children is seen in symptoms of reexperiencing the event, avoidance, and increased arousal in ways that go beyond the classic *DSM-IV* criteria. Social withdrawal, night terrors, separation anxiety, and a loss of previously learned skills can occur as a child's fear from an event produces a desire to retreat back to people and environments in which they have felt safe in the past. In the case of Mikail, trauma-related anxiety developed as a result of living in a war-torn region.

MIKAIL

Mikail was a ten-year-old boy who lived outside Sarajevo. He stayed with relatives while his parents relocated in the United States. Several months later when they were ready for Mikail to join them, the war intensified. His parents tried for a year to make contact with their relatives and to send money for his safe exit before they were finally able to be reunited. Mikail spoke very little to his parents about his experience. They soon observed, however, that he was having nightmares and difficulties sleeping. He appeared jumpy and was playing aggressively with other children. Therapy revealed that Mikail was having extensive dreams and nightmares of his relatives, killings, and warfare. He reported jumping when he heard loud noises that reminded him of the distant sound of bombings. He was uncomfortable looking at pictures of the home in Sarajevo and tried to avoid news reports of the fighting.

Other Anxiety Disorders

Although we have discussed the primary diagnoses of anxiety in children, there are several other conditions that warrant a brief review. Panic Attacks (PNA) and Panic Disorder (PD), characterized by brief recurrent feelings of fear accompanied by physiological symptoms, are not often seen in school-age children. Instances usually occur around a specific stressful event and are often in concert with other anxiety-related diagnosis, such as PTSD. Panic symptoms are more common in girls than in boys.

Although the incidence of this diagnosis is low for school-age children, case studies document its occurrence. At issue is the diagnostic criterion which states that the person experiences imminent fear or harm. Further, the person also must be able to envision or formulate negative outcomes from attacks. Some argue that, according to Piagetian stages of development, many school-age children have not yet developed the cognitive ability necessary to formulate these ideas and therefore cannot meet criteria. SAD is believed to be the childhood version of PNA and PD, as its behavioral descriptions are more age appropriate; this may account for the low frequency of panic diagnoses.

Generalized Anxiety Disorder (GAD) is another disorder that occurs infrequently in the school-age population. GAD also is sometimes diagnosed with PTSD in cases in which the behavioral symptoms of anxiety go beyond those of the arousal symptoms of PTSD and include worrying.

CO-MORBIDITY

Anxiety can coexist with and be related to a number of different disorders. In some cases, the presence of another psychiatric disorder can give rise to anxiety symptoms. Sometimes, it is difficult to ascertain which came first.

School-related difficulties such as learning disabilities and attention problems such as Attention Deficit Hyperactivity Disorder (ADHD) can lead to anxiety symptoms, particularly when a child is undiagnosed. A child's inability to perform as anticipated by parents and teachers can lead to frustration at school. This in turn can lead to anxiety and in some cases to school phobia. Academic testing that reveals these difficulties can often decrease the level of anxiety a child experiences, as she is given a concrete reason for her difficulties and can begin to manage them in a more appropriate way.

Children who have suffered a trauma can also present with anxiety symptoms beyond those of PTSD. Anxiety-driven behaviors such as worrying and oversensitivity are often associated with PTSD but can go beyond the conventional diagnostic criteria. Additionally, some behavior, though related to the traumatic event, may warrant a secondary diagnosis, as in the case that follows.

FRANK

Frank, a twelve-year-old Hispanic boy, was hit by a car while he was walking home from school. He sustained minor cuts and bruises, had no loss of consciousness, and was released from the hospital after one day. Upon returning home, Frank reported vague symptoms that initially kept him from attending school. After several months, Frank still complained of headaches and had not returned to school. Over the months following the accident, Frank isolated himself in his house. He would not go outside for fear that something might happen, and would not associate with any of his friends. He felt safest when he was with his parents and ventured from the house only if accompanied by one of them.

Depression is often associated with anxiety. As many as 69 percent of children with anxiety disorders also experience some depressive symptoms. These symptoms are often the result of the life changes that have occurred because of their anxiety. Isolation, repetitive behaviors, and need for the closeness of others can be very disruptive for a child as well as for his parents or guardians. In many cases, children are aware of what they are not able to do because of their anxiety and are mournful. In other cases, the predisposing event, such as the death of the grandfather in his sleep, can lead both to the child's fear of going to bed and to depression.

TREATMENT

Our treatment approach is based primarily on a cognitive-behavioral model but is informed by psychodynamic theory and technique. In this section, we discuss individual therapy and the techniques used, as well as play, group, and family therapy. We also review psychodynamic approaches and medication. Finally, we provide a guide to appropriate interventions.

Individual Therapy

Once you have completed your assessment, the next step is to set the stage for treatment by educating the child and parents about the specific anxiety disorder diagnosis. We explain the cognitive-behavioral conceptualization of anxiety and orient patients and families to the collaborative nature of the therapeutic relationship. This is followed by a discussion of the importance of exposure to feared stimuli and the necessity of the child's practicing his new skills between sessions.

When describing the cognitive-behavioral conceptualization of anxiety, we focus on the three ways in which anxiety is manifested: (1) bodily reactions, such as rapid heart rate, sweating hands, and dizziness; (2) cognitions or thoughts, such as "They'll make fun of me in class," or "If my mom leaves me, something bad will happen to her"; (3) actions or behaviors, such as avoiding feared situations or objects.

Treatment addresses the three manifestations of anxiety using a combination of cognitive and behavioral techniques. The following list presents a number of cognitive and behavioral techniques that are commonly used in the treatment of childhood anxiety.

- Exposure
- Contingency management (modification of antecedent and consequent events using operant principles such as reinforcement, extinction, and the like)
- Relaxation
- Modeling and role playing
- Cognitive techniques

Exposure Techniques. These techniques are the mainstay of treatment for most anxiety problems. The exposure can be conducted gradually, following a fear hierarchy of least to most anxiety provoking. Alternatively, you can employ prolonged and repeated exposure (flooding). Exposure techniques can also be conducted in vivo or by using visualization when it is impossible or impractical to return to or re-create the scene of the event. In our experience, in vivo exposure techniques tend to be more effective.

Contingency Management Techniques. These techniques are useful in most cases of childhood anxiety. They are derived from the principles of operant conditioning and are used to modify antecedent and consequent events that influence anxious behavior. They include such strategies as positive reinforcement, extinction, shaping, and punishment. The use of written contingency contracts can ensure that both the child and parents understand what is expected of them in the treatment plan. In the simplest form, you can use these strategies to encourage compliance with the treatment plan, for example, using rewards for following through with home exposure tasks. In some cases, however, they may be a central feature of the treatment. In many cases of childhood anxiety, there is inadvertent reinforcement of anxious behavior by parents and even teachers, as the following case illustrates.

KELLY

Kelly was a nine-year-old girl with separation anxiety and school avoidance. Kelly's difficulties initially presented as somatic complaints (headaches, stomachaches) that led to school absences. When she had complained of feeling ill, her parents would let her stay home, where she received attentive care from her mother and watched many of her favorite TV shows. Her teacher tried to be very flexible, dropping assignments off at her house (she lived in their neighborhood) and even shortening some of them because of her health problems.

Kelly's pediatrician, finding no medical explanation for her complaints and observing a fair amount of anxious behavior when Kelly's mother left the office to use the restroom, referred her for a psychological evaluation. The evaluation revealed that Kelly was very concerned about her mother's whereabouts, and she worried about her mother's and her own safety if they were separated. Her somatic complaints had become a vehicle for avoiding anxiety related to separations, a strategy that was being unwittingly reinforced by her parents and teacher. A central aspect of Kelly's treatment entailed working with the parents and teacher to alter their response to illness behavior and to increase their reinforcement of more adaptive behaviors. For example, when too "ill" to attend school, Kelly had to stay in her room and rest, with no TV. Her mother limited the amount of attention she received on these days. However, if Kelly attended a full day of school, she earned special privileges at home. Of course, modifying the behavioral contingencies was done in conjunction with teaching Kelly additional anxiety self-management strategies.

Relaxation Strategies. These strategies are valuable tools for managing anxiety. Generally, the child is taught to progressively relax the major muscle groups of the body by systematically tensing and releasing each muscle group. This enables her to perceive the differences between tense and relaxed states, which in turn enables her to learn to use the sensation of tension as a signal to relax. Children can also be taught cue-controlled relaxation, a process that involves a repeated association of a cue word of their choosing, such as "relax" or "calm," with the relaxed state. For example, when ten-year-old Katie began to feel anxious, which she described as "feeling like my body gets revved up," she would close her eyes, take a deep breath, and say the words "slow down" as she exhaled. There are a number of published relaxation scripts for children that are useful guides for therapists. When teaching relaxation, it is important to avoid conveying to the child that anxiety is bad and something to be avoided at all costs. Rather, the child should understand that relaxation is a tool to help him cope with anxiety so that intense anxiety no longer becomes a reason to engage in avoidant behavior.

Modeling. This technique involves demonstrating non-fearful behavior in the face of the feared stimulus, providing an opportunity for the child to observe and imitate appropriate behavior. Participant modeling entails interaction between the model and the child, with the model guiding the child's approach to the feared object or situation. Modeling was used in the case of Chris, a seven-year-old boy with an insect phobia. Following a process of gradual exposure, the therapist modeled appropriate behavior by handling insects (ants and spiders) while guiding Chris to do the same.

Cognitive Techniques. These techniques can be particularly useful when dealing with older children. In general, we tend to rely somewhat more on behavioral techniques for younger children because of the limits that cognitive development places on a young child's ability to identify and articulate what he is thinking in a particular situation. Philip Kendall describes the process of building a "cognitive coping template" that involves identifying and modifying maladaptive self-talk, along with building a new structure in which to view situations—a structure based on coping. The process is twofold: you first work with the child to remove characteristic misinterpretations of environmental events and then gradually and systematically build a frame of reference that includes strategies for coping.

The process is similar conceptually to cognitive therapy with adults, but you often need to be creative in order to make the concepts more tangible. For example, using cartoons with empty thought bubbles is an effective strategy. You ask the child to generate a variety of alternatives for what the character might be thinking in a situation, thus making the concept of cognitions and self-talk more accessible for the child.

Integrating Cognitive and Behavioral Techniques. Our approach to integrating cognitive and behavioral strategies draws on the work of Philip Kendall and his colleagues at Temple University. The skills training segment of the anxiety management program focuses on four basic skill areas: (1) awareness of the body's reactions to feelings and the physical symptoms of anxiety, (2) recognition and evaluation of cognitions or "self-talk" when anxious, (3) problem-solving skills (for example, modifying anxious self-talk and developing plans for coping), and (4) self-evaluation and reward for successful progress.

Following Kendall's model, we use the acronym FEAR as a way of helping children remember what to do when they feel anxious:

F: Feeling frightened? (recognizing physical symptoms of anxiety)

E: Expecting bad things to happen? (recognizing self-talk and what you are worried about)

A: Actions and attitudes that will help (different behaviors and coping statements the child can use in the anxiety-provoking situation, based on a problem-solving approach)

R: Results and rewards (self-evaluation and self-rewards)

The initial skills training portion of the treatment is followed by a practice phase. During this phase, the child is exposed to anxiety-provoking situations. Generally, the exposure follows a graded fear hierarchy, beginning with exposure to low-anxiety situations, followed by a gradual progression to situations that provoke higher anxiety.

The following case provides an example of an integrated cognitive-behavioral approach.

BRENDA

Brenda was a twelve-year-old girl who witnessed a robbery and shooting as she was coming out of her ballet class late one afternoon. She recognized that her heart rate went up when she approached the neighborhood where the robbery took place. She stopped going to ballet class, convincing herself that she could not dance well and did not like her teacher, and tried to avoid the area near the incident as well as anything related to ballet. She felt unsafe in the area and became upset when any of her family traveled in that part of town, particularly if it was late in the afternoon.

Brenda was taught relaxation techniques, which she used when she was exposed to situations or objects that reminded her of the event. She learned of the connection between her negative thoughts and beliefs and how they related to the accident, which led to more positive thoughts about dancing. She was able to identify that her negative feelings toward her teacher were related to feelings of being unprotected. Her negative thoughts and subsequent anxiety when a family member would leave the house were also addressed through an evaluation of her self-talk and through relaxation. Gradually, Brenda was exposed to the part of town where the incident took place and, eventually, to the place where she was standing when she witnessed the robbery and shooting.

Play Therapy

In some cases, the addition of the more traditional child therapy techniques of play and drawing can be useful. This is particularly the case when working with young children who have been exposed to a traumatic event. Young children involved in or exposed to a traumatic event can benefit from repeated play sessions in which they reenact the event with dolls and other toys. You can identify fears and cognitions in the play themes. Different scenarios of the event, authored and acted out by the child, help to reduce anxiety and aid the therapist in identifying additional fears or fantasies about the event.

Group Therapy

As with many disorders, anxiety disorders can be treated effectively in the group setting. For diagnoses such as OCD and PTSD, groups can provide a valuable forum for children to discuss their symptoms and experiences without feeling that they are "weird" or "crazy" (labels they fear may be applied to them if they were to discuss their feelings with peers at school). Social phobias, in particular, are very amenable to group therapy. The group experience allows children to work on their fears in a supportive environment with others struggling with similar issues. As with all anxiety disorders, you should thoroughly assess the nature of each child's anxiety prior to starting a group, considering the incidence of co-morbidity that can affect the progress of group treatment.

Some anxiety disorders, depending on how they present, are initially better addressed in individual therapy, with group therapy participation coming later in the treatment process. This is often particularly true in cases of PTSD in which the child's anxiety and experience are too personal to be initially shared in a group format.

Family Therapy

Family therapy is extremely important in the treatment of anxiety in school-age children because so much of their environment is in the hands of their parents or primary caretaker. It is important for parents to be allied with the therapist in supporting the therapeutic recommendations and treatment plan, as they are often responsible for carrying out rewards and facilitating gradual exposure to feared stimuli. Periodic sessions allow the parents to provide and receive feedback on the course of treatment and their role; parents also receive ongoing psychoeducation about the progress of therapy.

Family therapy is also valuable because, as mentioned earlier in the chapter, behavior changes in the child can often disrupt the family dynamics. In many cases the roles and behaviors of family members serve to support the anxiety in an attempt to alleviate other stressors, as we see in the following case example.

VINCENT

Seven-year-old Vincent was fearful of the dark, and he refused to go to school. Despite multiple attempts to institute treatment plans, Vincent's mother consistently made excuses for why they were not carried out. Morning hours were spent trying unsuccessfully to get Vincent to go to school, and evenings were spent in preparation for bedtime, which Vincent strongly resisted. Most nights, his mother stayed with him until he fell asleep, which often resulted in her falling asleep in his bed. With the commencement of family sessions, Vincent's parents revealed multiple difficulties in their marriage. In a private session with the parents, we identified that Vincent's anxiety kept distance between them. We discovered that the majority of the time when Dad was at home, Mom was attending to Vincent, which prevented them from addressing their own problems.

Psychodynamic Techniques

As we mentioned earlier, our approach to treatment relies greatly on a cognitive-behavioral model, but we also draw on psychodynamic theory and technique. It can be a challenge to blend the two approaches, and there is little in the literature that addresses integration of the two in the treatment of childhood anxiety. Many of our cases lend themselves to a straightforward cognitive-behavioral approach. However, for children and families with longer-standing and more severe psychopathology, or in situations where there is little progress, integration of psychodynamic theory and techniques can bridge the therapeutic gap that is harder to traverse with cognitive-behavioral techniques alone. The following case provides an example.

SUSAN

Susan was a nine-year-old girl with separation anxiety. She had been home schooled for a year because of her severe anxiety. Despite the therapist's (Collier's) best efforts at teaching Susan anxiety management skills and creating an appropriate behavioral plan, little progress was made. Each new suggestion made to Susan's mother, Lisa, for management of the problem was met with a list of reasons why that plan was unlikely to work. Lisa was always apologetic about failing to follow through, and appeared to expect the therapist to get angry. Getting nowhere fast, I decided to suspend pursuit of the cognitive-behavioral treatment plan temporarily while I took the time to explore the meaning of progress to Susan and Lisa.

It quickly became clear that, although Lisa wanted her daughter to be able to function normally, she had her own anxiety about being without Susan. She viewed Susan as fragile and unable to tolerate intense anxiety but also viewed herself that way. She was most at ease when Susan was near. Some of Lisa's anxiety about being alone dated back to the sudden and traumatic death of her own father in a car accident that occurred when she was nine, the same age as Susan. Lisa's mother, who was very involved in the lives of her daughter and granddaughter, was a rather domineering woman. Lisa frequently felt that she was unable to live up to her mother's expectations, and she perceived her mother as getting angry with her when this occurred. Exploring the meaning of the situation for Lisa and the way it affected treatment and her relationship with the therapist was the key to eventual therapeutic success.

Psychopharmacology

Medications have proven useful in the treatment of many children with anxiety disorders. We have found it to be beneficial for children whose symptoms have failed to respond adequately to therapy. Medication can also be helpful when severe anxiety interferes with a child's ability to engage in therapy effectively. Some children are overwhelmed by their symptoms to such an extent that their daily life is significantly altered. This is sometimes the case in children diagnosed with PTSD who become isolated, have repeated temper outbursts, refuse to go to school, and are frequently tearful.

Both anti-anxiety and antidepressant medications are used to treat anxiety disorders. Tricyclic antidepressants are effective for children with selected types of anxiety disorders. Selective serotonin reuptake inhibitor (SSRI) antidepressants are an additional treatment option and exhibit few side effects. Anti-anxiety medications such as benzodiazepines are also effective for a number of anxiety disorders. Unlike some anti-anxiety medications, however, antidepressants do not have abuse potential. As with any medication, you need to conduct appropriate baseline laboratory studies and regularly monitor drug levels and side effects. Table 2.2 shows the preferred medications for each disorder.

Table 2.2
Medications Used to Treat Anxiety Disorders

Diagnosis	*Medications*	*Comments*
Obsessive-Compulsive Disorder	Clomipramine Fluxetine Sertraline	All are primary medications used
Separation Anxiety and school phobia	Imipramine Alprazolam Chlordiazepoxide Clomazepam	Imipramine most often
Generalized Anxiety Disorder with Childhood Onset	Buspirone Clomazepam Alprazolam Fluoxetine	Buspirone and Fluoxetine most often
Panic Disorder	Imipramine Desipramine Clomazepam Alprazolam Fluoxetine	Fluoxetine and Imipramine commonly used
Childhood-onset Social Phobia	Buspirone Alprazolam Fluoxetine	All have been used; Fluoxetine may be more helpful
PTSD	Imipramine Buspirone	Imipramine most often

Choosing Interventions

Decisions about which techniques or interventions to use and when to use them are driven both by the case formulation for that particular patient and the nature of her specific anxiety disorder. The case formulation, key in any successful course of therapy, provides a synthesis of the factors hypothesized to underlie a patient's problems. It is this understanding of the influence of such factors as cognitions, coping style, family dynamics, stage of development, and so on that suggests priorities for treatment and guides the timing and choice of interventions.

The specific anxiety disorder will also shape your selection of interventions. For example, although relaxation approaches are commonly incorporated in the treatment for most of the anxiety disorders, they tend to be ineffective for most patients with OCD. Cognitive strategies also tend to add little to the treatment of OCD. The most effective nonpharmacological treatment for OCD is exposure and response prevention. In this technique, the patient is exposed to the feared object or situation and is instructed to gradually increase the length of time during which he refrains from all ritualistic (anxiety-reducing) behavior.

For most phobias, gradual progression during exposure to the feared object or situation is the treatment of choice. However, for school phobia that is secondary to Separation Anxiety Disorder, it is often best to move much more quickly in your efforts to get the child back in the school setting, particularly if the onset of the school avoidance is recent. Prompt return to school is essential, because the longer a child is out of school, the more difficult it is to get her back. School phobias of long-standing duration may be more resistant to a more rapid return and require a more gradual approach.

Other instances in which the anxiety diagnosis may drive your selection of interventions include the use of groups for social anxiety and the use of play techniques for the treatment of PTSD in the young child.

Managed Care

Managed care influences much of our work these days. Most of our patients have a limited number of sessions each year, and some managed care organizations require updates every few sessions to review progress toward the therapeutic goals.

Fortunately, cognitive-behavioral approaches to the treatment of anxiety disorders generally lend themselves well to a managed care framework. You can easily define behavioral goals, you employ specific interventions, and the child's progress in many cases is relatively rapid.

Of course, not all cases fit neatly into this framework. Some of your more complex cases that involve, for example, a problem of long-standing duration or co-morbid diagnoses, may require more than the allotted number of sessions. In these situations you are faced with educating the reviewer about the unique issues in the cases, clearly outlining why more sessions are needed and what you plan to do in those sessions.

Offering to send the case reviewer a written summary can be helpful. If further sessions are initially denied, inquire about an appeals process or ask to speak to the reviewer's supervisor or the medical director. Sometimes a child's pediatrician can be an ally and can "go to bat" for you.

Finally, it is always important to discuss with the parents the parameters of their coverage and to design a treatment plan that can reasonably be accomplished in the allotted time. You may not be able to address every psychodynamic issue in a case, but you can still effect important behavioral changes (such as returning to school) that will have a positive impact on a child's quality of life.

Anxiety disorders affect a significant proportion of children. As we have discussed, through careful assessment and diagnosis you can usually achieve a significant decrease or resolution of symptoms. Early detection and treatment can not only provide relief and improve functioning but can also provide the child and the

parents with valuable tools for dealing with future anxiety-pro-
ducing situations and events.

NOTES

P. 34, *Studies have found that as many as 17 percent:* Costello, E. J., Stouthamer-
Loeber, M., & DeRosier, M. (1993). *Continuity and change in psychopathol-
ogy from childhood to adolescence.* Paper presented at Annual Meeting of
Society for Researcher in Child and Adolescent Psychopathology, Santa
Fe, NM.

P. 34, *determine whether anxiety represents a transient reaction:* Hayward, C., &
Collier, J. A. (1996). Anxiety disorders. In H. Steiner (Ed.), *Treating adolescents.* San Francisco: Jossey-Bass.

P. 35, *medical evaluation is warranted:* Hayward, C., & Collier, J. A. (1996). *ibid.*

P. 35, *it can be difficult to differentiate the contribution of genetics:* Hayward, C.,
& Collier, J. A. (1996). *ibid.*

P. 36, *Other stressors:* Hayward, C., & Collier, J. A. (1996). *ibid.*

P. 41, *the most common childhood compulsions:* Swedo, S. E., Rapoport, J. L.,
Leonard, H., Lenane, M., & Cheslow, D. (1989). Obsessive-compulsive
disorder in children and adolescents: Clinical phenomenology of 70 consecutive cases. *Archives of General Psychiatry, 46*(4), 335–341.

P. 42, *They appear to be more common in boys:* Swedo, S. E., Rapoport, J. L.,
Leonard, H., Lenane, M., & Cheslow, D. (1989). *ibid;* Last, C., & Strauss, C.
(1989). Obsessive-compulsive disorder in childhood. *Journal of Anxiety Disorders, 3,* 295–301.

P. 43, *SAD occurs most frequently . . . found in girls:* Last, C., Francis, G., Hersen,
M., Kazdin, A. E., & Strauss, C. C. (1987). Separation anxiety and school
phobia: A comparison using DSM-III criteria. *American Journal of Psychiatry, 144,* 653–657.

P. 43, *A diagnosis of Specific Phobia:* American Psychiatric Association. (1994).
Diagnostic and statistical manual of mental disorders (4th ed., p. 405). Washington, DC: Author.

P. 44, *Debra Biedel identified a broad range of stressful social encounters:* Biedel, D.
(1995). Social phobia. In J. March (Ed.), *Anxiety disorders in children and adolescents* (pp. 181–211). New York: Guilford Press.

P. 44, *Jerome Kagan and his colleagues at Harvard reported:* Biederman, J., Rosen-
baum, J. F., Chaloff, J., & Kagan, J. (1995). Behavioral inhibition as a risk

factor for anxiety disorders. In J. March (Ed.), *Anxiety disorders in children and adolescents* (pp. 61–81). New York: Guilford Press.

P. 44, *"I stopped talking . . . never told anyone"*: Goben, J. (1996, June 9). A little help from her friends. *San Francisco Chronicle*. Reprinted by permission.

P. 46, *the DSM-IV classification of a traumatic event*: American Psychiatric Association. (1994). *ibid.*

P. 46, *Social withdrawal, night terrors*: Scheeringa, M. S., Zeanah, C. H., Drell, M. J., & Larrien, J. A. (1995). Two approaches to the diagnosis of post-traumatic stress disorder in infancy and early childhood. *Journal of the American Academy of Child and Adolescent Psychiatry, 34*(2), 191–200.

P. 47, *other anxiety-related diagnoses, such as PTSD*: King, N. J., Ollendick, T. H., & Mattis, S. G. (1994). Pain in children and adolescents: Normative and clinical studies. *Australian Psychologist, 29*(2), 89–93.

P. 47, *many school-age children . . . cannot meet criteria*: Nelles, W. B., & Barlow, D. H. (1988). Do children panic? *Clinical Psychology Review, 8,* 259–272.

P. 49, *As many as 69 percent of children with anxiety disorders*: Brady, E., & Kendall, P. (1992). Comorbidity of anxiety and depression in children and adolescents. *Psychological Bulletin, 111,* 244–255.

P. 49, *a discussion of the importance of exposure*: Hayward, C., & Collier, J. A. (1996). *ibid;* Silverman, W. K., Ginsburg, G. S., & Kurtines, W. M. (1995). Clinical issues in treating children with anxiety and phobic disorders. *Cognitive and Behavioral Practice, 2*(1), 93–117.

P. 49, *the three ways in which anxiety is manifested*: Hayward, C., & Collier, J. A. (1996). *ibid;* Silverman, W. K., Ginsburg, G. S., & Kurtines, W. M. (1995). *ibid.*

P. 52, *use the sensation of tension . . . relax*: Kendall, P. C., Chansky, T. E., Freidman, M., Kim, R., Kortlander, E., Sessa, F. M., & Siqueland, L. (1991). Treating anxiety disorders in children and adolescents. In P. C. Kendall (Ed.), *Child and adolescent therapy*. New York: Guilford Press.

P. 52, *such as "relax" or "calm"*: Kendall, P. C, Chansky, T. E., Freidman, M., Kim, R., Kortlander, E., Sessa, F. M., & Siqueland, L. (1991). *ibid.*

P. 52, *two relaxation scripts*: Koeppen, A. S. (1974). Relaxation training for children. *Elementary School Guidance and Counseling, 9,* 14–21; Ollendick, T. H., & Cerny, J. A. (1981). *Clinical behavior therapy with children*. New York: Plenum Press.

P. 52, *the child should understand . . . engage in avoidant behavior*: Hayward, C., & Collier, J. A. (1996). *ibid.*

P. 53, *"cognitive coping template"*: Kendall, P. C., Chansky, T. E., Freidman, M., Kim, R., Kortlander, E., Sessa, F. M., & Siqueland, L. (1991). *ibid.*

P. 53, *Our approach to integrating:* Kendall, P. C., Chansky, T. E., Freidman, M., Kim, R., Kortlander, E., Sessa, F. M., & Siqueland, L. (1991). *ibid.*

P. 60, *which techniques or interventions to use:* Hayward, C., & Collier, J. A. (1996). *ibid.*

P. 60, *The case formulation:* Hayward, C., & Collier, J. A. (1996). *ibid;* Wilkes, T. C. R., Belsher, G., Rush, A. J., Frank, E., and Associates (1994). *Cognitive therapy for depressed adolescents.* New York: Guilford Press.

P. 60, *the longer a child is out of school:* Black, B. (1995). Separation anxiety disorder and panic disorder. In J. S. March (Ed.), *Anxiety disorders in children and adolescents.* New York: Guilford Press.

3

DEPRESSION

James Lock

ALEX

Alex was a quiet and sensitive eight-year-old boy who had always been a good student. He was quite hard on himself and always thought he could do better. He was very close to both his parents and had a history of worrying a lot when they were away. When his family moved from the Midwest to the West Coast, however, Alex began to have more problems. His mother began working, and he started a new school where other children teased him for being a "nerd" and a "mama's boy."

At first Alex tried to ignore these taunts, but over time he began to avoid going to school. He complained of headaches and stomachaches, and of being very tired. When he did go to school, he did poorly. His grades dropped from A's to C's and D's. At home he began to whine and complain. He became increasingly needy. He fought more with his little sister and began to have trouble sleeping. He began to argue more about any requests his parents made of him. His mother noticed that he was looking skinny and took him to his pediatrician for an evaluation.

The pediatrician found no medical problems, but noted that he was not gaining weight as the doctor had expected. When the doctor asked Alex if he was sad, Alex admitted that he was and began to cry. "I'm a dummy and I'm a bad boy." He said, "I just want to go to sleep and not wake up."

As a child and adolescent psychiatrist working in an academic setting, I see many children who are depressed. I have treated children in a variety of programs, including inpatient, outpatient, and day treatment. I work with children and their families using a number of treatment approaches including medication and individual, family, and group therapy. School-age children with depression, I have found, are often the most difficult to identify, because people are reluctant to believe children at this age can be depressed. Once in treatment, however, school-age children are quite responsive to a range of treatments. There is a special pleasure in working with this age group because of the developmental characteristics of the period. The children's wish to understand rules and mostly follow them, to use fantasy and play to work out their problems, and to use adults to mediate their internal conflicts distinguish them from both younger children and adolescents. These characteristics make the use of play therapy and family therapy particularly rewarding and often successful with this population.

Not too many years ago, many people believed that children under the age of twelve did not suffer from problems with depression. Now, however, we know depressive symptoms begin as early as infancy. Studies of seriously deprived infants in World War II foundling homes, for example, showed that some infants became withdrawn and refused to eat, failed to develop, and eventually died. They resembled in almost every aspect the clinical picture of melancholic depression in adults.

In this chapter, I focus on treating depression in children who are between the ages of five and twelve. About 2 percent of these school-age children are depressed. Most of them are not identified and do not receive treatment, including those who we know are at greater risk. For example, studies of pediatric medical patients have demonstrated that between 7 and 30 percent of hospitalized children suffer from depression, but most of them are never treated.

DIFFERENTIAL DIAGNOSIS

When I am considering diagnosing a child with depression, I review the risk factors that increase the possibility of a child developing this disorder. If there is a family history of depression, the risk is approximately 10 to 13 percent. Rates are higher for fraternal (dizygotic) twins and highest for identical (monozygotic) twins. A child's risk for a Major Depression is also increased if there is a history of parental alcoholism or death before a child is thirteen years old. Chronic illness, stressful life events such as trauma and abuse, and family factors such as divorce, marital discord, and ongoing parent-child conflicts also increase the risk. Combination with other risk factors compounds the possibility that the child will develop a depressive illness.

Many other disorders may resemble one of the clinical syndromes of depression. An important part of my initial assessment is to make sure I have not mistaken any of the following disorders for a depression.

Adjustment Disorders

An adjustment disorder is a response or adjustment to a change or stress. The hallmark of adjustment disorders is the clear identification of a specific stress or significant change that corresponds in time to the onset of a depressed mood and a decreased ability to work, play, or study. Children may experience these kinds of adjustment problems in the context of many situations, such as a family move, parental separation or divorce, or an injury or illness. Supportive intervention is usually enough to assist children and their families during adjustment periods.

It is easy to mistake an adjustment disorder for a depression, but it is also easy to miss a depression. An example of this is the case of Alex, the eight-year-old I described at the beginning of the chapter. When the school counselor referred him to me, I thought at first that he was having trouble adjusting to his new environment, but when I was able to get a thorough history, I found that his difficulties with depression had begun a month or more before moving. I had to adjust my treatment plan to make it a more aggressive one that addressed Alex's depression as well as his adjustment problems.

Normal Bereavement

The death of someone close to a child may lead to normal bereavement processes. Children may have difficulty sleeping, become more withdrawn, and show regressive behavior for a two- to three-week period following such a loss. Sometimes bereavement does lead to a Major Depression when grieving becomes extended and the symptoms or behaviors more pronounced, or if the child's self-esteem or self-image is negatively affected. I do not automatically assume that a child who has experienced a significant loss has a depression, but my experience has been that people more commonly fail to identify a depression after a loss than vice versa.

Separation Anxiety Disorder

As discussed in Chapter Two, this disorder is associated with a child's fear of separation from someone to whom she is attached. The symptoms include sadness, excessive worry, sleep problems, feeling physically ill, and trying to stay home, but only in the context of separation from the attachment figure. Usual intervention includes psychotherapeutic work with both the child and family. Depression occurs as an independent condition in a significant proportion of these children.

In my experience with school-age children, there sometimes is an overlap between Major Depression and Separation Anxiety Disorder. If this overlap isn't recognized, the child is unlikely to respond well to treatment. For example, I treated a nine-year-old girl whose outpatient psychiatrist was at his wit's end because she continued to be depressed after trials of both medication and psychotherapy. When she was admitted to our hospital, she was unable to separate from her mother—and her mother was unable to separate from her. Although the girl was depressed, her symptoms worsened when her mother was absent or did not call. Only when I also addressed her Separation Anxiety Disorder through family treatment was I able to make progress with her depression.

TYPES OF DEPRESSION

There are several types of depression that are recognized in the current diagnostic system. Although my focus in this chapter is on Major Depression, the most common type of depression, it is important to distinguish between the types of depression to ensure that any treatment you undertake is the right one for the child.

Major Depression

According to the *DSM-IV*, there is little difference between children, adolescents, or adults in terms of how Major Depression looks. For children to be diagnosed with Major Depression they must have a depressed or irritable mood or a decreased interest in previously pleasurable activities for two consecutive weeks. They must no longer participate in school or social activities as before. In addition, they must have four of the following symptoms:

- Sleep disturbance
- Weight or appetite disturbance
- Problems in concentration
- Suicidal ideation or thoughts of death
- Observable increased or decreased activity

- Fatigue or loss of energy
- Feelings of being worthless
- Inappropriate guilt

Dysthymia

Dysthymia is diagnosed when a child has a depressed or irritable mood for more days than not for about a year. The difference between Dysthymia and Major Depression is related to both the severity and persistence of the symptoms. Major Depression is more severe but remits after a few months. Dysthymia has less pronounced symptoms, but they are chronic. It is important to note that Dysthymia is not a "little" Major Depression. It is a pattern of lowered mood that results in longer-term chronic depressive behaviors.

The *DSM-IV* describes Dysthymia in children as consisting of a depressed mood for most of the day for most days for a year. In addition, children must have at least two of the following symptoms:

- Poor appetite or overeating
- Insomnia or hypersomnia
- Low energy or fatigue
- Low self-esteem
- Poor concentration or difficulty making decisions
- Feelings of hopelessness

Children must not have suffered a Major Depression within a year and never have had a manic episode. These symptoms must not result from a medical condition or from the use of alcohol or drugs. Together these symptoms must result in impairment of social, school, or interpersonal relations.

The chronic and persistent nature of the symptoms may actually lead to a Major Depression—a so-called double depression.

In this case, treatment of the depression is often protracted and more difficult, as there is less likely to be a remission of all symptoms with the passing of the Major Depression. Chronic feelings like those associated with Major Depression can lead to a depressive pattern of interacting with others and chronic problems with schoolwork, and to hopelessness about the possibility of change in the future.

I have seen Dysthymia mistaken for a temperamental condition or a character or personality style, or dismissed as "moodiness." Such mistakes lead to inadequate treatment that can result in poor school, social, and interpersonal functioning for a lifetime.

Bipolar Affective Disorder

Bipolar Disorder affects about 1 percent of the population and is considered to be inherited—though exactly how this occurs is not well understood. About 20 percent of Bipolar Disorder is thought to have its onset during childhood and adolescence, but it is often not diagnosed until much later because of the mixture of symptoms that characterize the illness.

Bipolar Disorder in children is often diagnosed as ADHD, Oppositional Defiant Disorder, or Major Depression. At least part of the reason for this has to do with how the illness usually begins. In young children, the full syndrome for depression may not be easily seen. Irritability, disobedience, lability, and peer and school problems are instead seen as the result of family problems, temperament, or disciplinary problems—which indeed they are in many cases. However, the possibility of nascent bipolar illness should be considered in cases where the usual interventions for these disorders and problems fail or when there is a strong family history of affective illness.

Because Bipolar Disorder is seldom diagnosed in school-age children, I do not discuss treatment for this disorder in this chapter. Sometimes a depressed child will later develop a bipolar illness. In this case, the therapeutic treatment, other than medications, would be the same as I would use to treat Major Depression.

Cyclothymia

Cyclothymia is a disorder similar to, but not as severe as, Bipolar Disorder. As the name suggests, there is a cycling of moods in this disorder as in Bipolar Disorder, but the severity and chronicity of the mood changes are different.

The *DSM-IV* requires that the person experiences hypomania—an expansive high mood that does not lead to impaired judgment or severe behavioral problems—numerous times over a one-year period, as well as experiencing periods of numerous depressive symptoms that don't meet the criteria for a Major Depression. In children there can be no longer than a two-month period without mood problems during a two-year period, and the child cannot have experienced manic episodes or a Major Depression during the first two years of the mood cycles. These mood cycles must lead to a disturbance in social, work, or family relations and cannot be due to a physical illness or be secondary to the use of alcohol, drugs, or medications. Of course the child cannot be suffering from a psychotic or other mood disorder. Cyclothymia, like Bipolar Disorder, is seldom diagnosed in children, so I do not discuss treatment for this mood disorder in this chapter.

ASSESSMENT OF MAJOR DEPRESSION

Assessment of young children for Major Depression requires an understanding of physical, emotional, and psychological variables. In this section, I describe how I use a developmental approach in evaluating children for depression. Specifically, I describe the elements of the clinical presentation and mental status examination that you need to pay special attention to when evaluating young children for depressive disorders.

Clinical Presentation

As I implied earlier, the *DSM-IV* provides little guidance on how Major Depression appears in different age groups. Major Depression in children and adults does present in a comparable manner at least some of the time. On the other hand, developmental variables may also complicate and limit the utility of some aspects of diagnostic criteria. The physical changes in the brain and body of a child in terms of neurochemistry and hormonal environment differ from that in adults, and the impact of these biological differences and changes is not well understood.

School-age children tend to be rather concrete in their thinking; they present subjective emotional states, and depressed states in particular, in terms they can understand—such as pain, aches, and other somatic complaints. Symptomatic expression in children and adolescents is limited to a certain extent by developmental capacities. Very young children have trouble identifying their feeling states. Language is not a reliable tool, and thus certain diagnostic elements are difficult to assess, thereby making it more difficult to document all the elements required to make the diagnosis.

Children are also more labile and variable in their emotional states. This makes it difficult to make an accurate diagnosis on the basis of a single interview. It may well take several interviews over a several-day period to get an overall and consistent picture of the mood and affect of a particular child. Children can also express their depression with increased irritability, which can be confusing because this can appear to be an oppositional or behavioral problem. But it is important to remember that children have a more limited repertoire of symptom expression, and in some cases this irritability speaks to their inner discontent and difficulty.

The average age of onset of Major Depression in school-age children is between eight and fourteen. In general, children of all age groups present with a depressed mood, problems with concentration, insomnia, and some degree of suicidal ideation.

But with increasing age there is a decline in depressed appearance and somatic complaints in general, and an increasing prevalence of anhedonia, diurnal variation in symptoms, hopelessness, psychomotor retardation, and delusions. In school-age children, somatic complaints, agitation, single-voice auditory hallucinations, and co-morbid anxiety disorders and phobias are common presenting symptoms.

In order to assess a school-age child you should attend to nonverbal communication such as facial expression and body posture, and observe for listlessness, withdrawal, and weepiness. A history of weight loss, sleep disturbances, and refusing to eat is common. The child's school performance deteriorates and he may drop out of favorite activities. Although suicidal thoughts do occur in young children, actual suicidal behavior is more associated with child abuse and neglect and with exposure to violence and to suicidal adults.

Mental Status Examination

On mental status examination, clinically depressed children will look sad; they are tearful, have slowed movements and a monotone voice, and speak in a hopeless and despairing manner. Depressed children will describe themselves in negative terms, such as "I'm dumb," "I'm a bad girl," and "Nobody cares about me." The child may have somatic complaints, such as headaches and stomachaches. In later childhood, depression will more often include reports of lowered self-esteem and self-reports of disappointment with themselves, apathy, irritability, and anxiety increase. School-age children are able to be interviewed about their emotions and feeling states; they often give information of which their parents are unaware about sadness, sleep disturbances, and suicidal thoughts.

Because depression does run in families, I am concerned about parental reporting of symptoms in their children. They may overreport out of their own depressive and negative worldview or underreport because of self-preoccupation and decreased concern about things around them.

MEDICATION

I use biological, psychological, and social interventions in my treatment of children with depressive disorders. Sometimes emphasis may fall more on one kind of intervention than another in a particular case, but in every case the child is considered in the context of the family, school, and cultural environments. These variables are critical to successful intervention with children and cannot be ignored.

Evaluation

As a child psychiatrist, I am often asked to evaluate a depressed child for a medication trial of antidepressants. I think it is important for nonpsychiatrists to understand what goes into such evaluations: when children and parents talk to you about their experiences, you can better appreciate what likely occurred.

I begin a medication evaluation by having a frank discussion with the family about our limited knowledge of antidepressant use in children. I tell them that a variety of such medications have been tried with children. Only recently have carefully conducted studies shown that active medication is more beneficial than placebo. This is not to say that medications don't help some children with depression—this is not at all the case—but I need to thwart expectations about a "magic pill" to solve all the problems a child is having.

Next, I discuss the range of current antidepressants, their respective side effects, and why I might recommend one over another in a particular case. Such variables as past allergies and cardiac, kidney, or liver problems are common considerations. Family history and particular side effects are always additional important concerns.

For reasons that are not entirely clear, some patients, adult or child, respond better to one medication over another. In addition, each medication has significant side effects and risks associated with it; if you are a psychiatrist, the decision about which medication to use and how to monitor it is an important one.

Proper medication management over the long term can help prevent the number and severity of depressive episodes. This will lead to better overall emotional and psychosocial functioning.

Consent

In my office, I always go over a written consent form with the parent and the child if she is old enough to play a role in the process. I speak in everyday language and explain the most common side effects of the medication. I usually ask both parent and child to sign it. Experience has shown me that children do not like to take medications of any kind, and drugs that they feel will affect their mind or feelings are particularly repugnant. They often experience medications as intrusive.

For the school-age child there is considerable peer pressure to be just like everyone else, and they may feel that they are different from and inferior to their peers if they take "pills." One depressed boy needed to take a dose of medicine during the lunch hour at school but repeatedly "forgot" to go to the nurse's office to get the pill. When I asked him about it he said, "I don't want to take pills at school. All the kids will tease me," expressing his anxiety about how he will be perceived by his peers. In fact, none of his schoolmates knew he was taking medication, but even the thought that they might find out was enough to make him cautious.

Managed Care

In today's environment of managed health care, I have experienced increased pressure to prescribe antidepressants for children without my conducting a thorough evaluation. I think it is imperative that all of us working with children do not succumb to a standard that puts children at risk for inappropriate care. When I have prescribed medication, I sometimes have difficulty getting approval for sufficient visits to monitor it safely. This can put psychiatrists and other mental health providers at odds with one another because both need to see a child within a schedule of insufficient coverage. In these instances, I try to develop a team approach that facilitates the overall best care of the child. Thus I may depend on some monitoring of behavioral responses from therapists, or at times a psychotherapy visit may have to be missed in order to monitor or adjust a medication.

When you refer a depressed child for a medication evaluation, be sure that the person you refer to is a board certified, board eligible child psychiatrist. Also make sure they are willing to continue monitoring the medication while you continue as the primary therapist. These basic guidelines will help you ensure that your patient is receiving appropriate treatment.

Compliance Problems

The specific issue of medication compliance usually affects all of us on a treatment team. If a child does not take medications as prescribed, therapists are likely to note difficulties in their psychotherapeutic work. It is also true that everyone can be a part of the solution to medication compliance problems.

I use the process of sharing information about the limitations of medications and signing the consent form as a way to establish a sense of respect for the child that I hope will help with compliance problems down the road. When I start a medication, I spend a great deal of time enlisting the child in the process by helping him identify what changes or gains he hopes to achieve as a result of taking the antidepressant. Many times these goals are not the ones I might set, but I find that by tracking them, I increase compliance and understanding of a particular child's struggles with depression. I often make a checklist of these goals and go over them with the child during subsequent medication visits.

Children from five to twelve may strongly resist taking medicine because of side effects, especially sleepiness and at times fuzzy-headedness, and because of the need for frequent visits to check blood level. Younger children often fear blood draws and resent them greatly. Also, because they are developmentally still concrete in their thinking, children often have trouble believing that they are still ill; they may discontinue their medications when they start to feel better, not realizing that they need to continue taking it. This often leads to a resurgence of their symptoms and more problems at home and school as a result. Individual therapy can help support children as well as help to increase compliance by way of encouraging the development of insight and understanding about their illness.

If you are working with children who are noncompliant on their medications, you can help the psychiatrist by providing regular information on the clinical status of the child. You may well be the first to suspect difficulties and alert the psychiatrist of your observations. Once the problem has been identified, you can support improved compliance by helping to discover the underlying causes for the noncompliant behavior and by developing strategies to address it.

Medications are not a panacea, and often the wish to have a quick fix with a pill can undermine other aspects of treatment. I often find myself helping other clinicians understand these limits. So although medications can be helpful in many cases, I find getting them started, continuing them in the face of side effects, and dealing with unrealistic expectations about their efficacy to be constant hazards.

PSYCHODYNAMIC AND SOCIAL APPROACHES

I seldom find the biological approach alone sufficient for treating depressed children. Most often, unless it is a clinically severe depression, I start with therapy, and if this proves to be inadequate, I then consider a medication trial.

Many of the issues associated with childhood depression can be seen as a part of childhood development. Difficulty in mastering developmental hurdles for whatever reason can lead to depression. I use a combination of individual, family, group, and cognitive approaches. As a starting point, I try to determine the developmental issues and how they may be contributing to the depression. However, I have found that there is a difference in my work with younger school-age children—ages five to eight years old—compared to my work with school-age children on the verge of adolescence. I therefore divide my discussion accordingly.

Younger School-Age Children (Five- to Eight-Year-Olds)

I will discuss my treatment of Andrew to illustrate how I use these various forms of therapy to help depressed children in the younger age group.

ANDREW

Andrew was a six-year-old boy referred to my office because of behavioral problems at school and home. His mother brought him in and reported that Andrew had been an ideal baby and toddler. She said he began to have minor problems with demanding and clinging behaviors after the birth of his younger brother about a year ago. However, he had more recently begun to eat poorly and had lost weight. His mother noted that these changes were associated with the occurrence of repeated absences of his father from home over the past several months. Andrew's teacher had called to tell her that he wasn't paying attention in school and cried easily when things didn't go exactly his way. His schoolmates called him "baby," and the teacher reported that he gave up easily on his schoolwork. At home Andrew had difficulty sleeping and often came to his mother's bed at night. He had multiple somatic complaints every week, including headaches and stomachaches. He threw tantrums over very trivial upsets.

Andrew's mother was worried about her son and had taken him to the pediatrician, who found nothing physically wrong with him and suggested that his problems might be emotional. Reluctantly, Andrew's mother accepted the suggestion that she call me for an appointment. Still, she postponed bringing Andrew in until he said he wanted to die.

On mental status examination, Andrew was a tall and attractive boy who looked physically older than six. He had a serious expression, and he seldom smiled or looked at me. He complained of being sad and claimed he couldn't play sports. He said he was "dumb" and felt that no one liked him. He said he "hated" his brother.

Individual Therapy. With school-age children it's important to make the therapeutic work fit into their experience as much as possible. Because behavior of school-age children is concerned with self-regulation and group cohesion, I try to make my therapeutic work responsive to this need for external structure. I do this by setting the therapeutic frame in terms they can appreciate and by using games as a method for structuring our interaction. My emphasis in these games is on emotional expression—either enhancement of repressed emotions or containment of volatile ones. Because this takes place within a "game" it is safer for the child to explore feelings.

School-age children remain competitive and aggressive but develop more socially acceptable ways of managing these impulses through the use of fantasy and games designed to help develop skills in game playing. School-age children also use fantasy so that they can explore alternatives without taking overt action. I therefore encourage the use of imaginative play to explore alternatives and unacceptable feelings. In addition, mastery of basic skills is fundamental to school-age children, so I often incorporate some work projects—such as constructing models or making something—into the therapeutic activity. I choose projects that lend themselves to joint work so that I can increase my rapport with more resistant children.

Individual sessions with Andrew started immediately after the evaluation. Play therapy sessions began with structured games such as checkers and Battleship. Andrew was initially overly competitive, and he struggled with impulses to cheat. His only pleasure was in winning overall. Interpretations of this as anger and frustration with his little brother and schoolmates tempered his behavior only moderately. However, these games did serve a positive function by helping to establish a routine structure for our sessions.

Andrew began to improve more when we began work on building things together while we talked. As time went by, we built a birdhouse that he took home and filled with birdseed to "take care of the birds." I interpreted this to him as a way he could take care of something smaller than him and in a way that he wished to be taken care of. Andrew tolerated interpretations of his need for support and wishes to combat dependency, and increasingly accepted and acknowledged his anger at his father for being away so often.

Andrew's depression improved because he learned important things through his play therapy. Perhaps most important, he learned that he needed and deserved to be taken care of by his parents—in other words, that he was not worthless. In addition, he mastered some of his worries about being replaced by his little brother that had resulted in aggressive and competitive feelings at school in his play sessions. I say "mastered" because Andrew did not really gain insight into his envy and anxiety so much as develop a way to manage them. In his case, this management was represented by Andrew's developing his own nurturing capacities for the birds. Instead of using more primitive aggressive and violent behaviors to manage his feelings, he developed the capacity to use this more age-appropriate and successful strategy.

The aim of play therapy for depression in school-age children is not insight but mastery. The structure is play, not words. The outcome is behavioral change, not personality change. So when designing a treatment plan for school-age children that involves play therapy, you should set goals that reflect this age-appropriate outcome. I have heard therapists say they intend to increase the insight of an eight-year-old child into the origins of her depression, but this is really not helpful. The eight-year-old needs to learn ways to manage her feelings more effectively, and this means, for this age group at least, that you may be the only person who perceives the play as addressing in an abstract way the core issues involved in the depression.

Today we all need to be aware of the management of health care resources. I work with utilization reviewers from various managed care companies from the outset. I develop a treatment plan that includes all the dimensions of treatment that I feel are critical to a successful outcome. I try to predict the approximate number of sessions I will need to see the child and family. I also set goals for treatment that are understandable for the reviewers of such a plan. For example, in Andrew's case, I told the reviewers that Andrew would likely require weekly individual treatment for three to six months and that if he did not respond in that time, I would reevaluate the plan. If he was doing better, I might cut back on sessions; if he was doing worse, I might increase the number of sessions. I determined that the goals of his treatment would be an improvement in mood, improved sleep and appetite, and improved school functioning. The reviewers found this plan agreeable, and I was able to proceed with the treatment I described.

Family Therapy. Family work followed closely behind the individual work with Andrew. It was difficult to get the entire family together because of the father's work schedule, but this difficulty quickly allowed us to identify it as an issue. When the family did get together, it was clearly difficult for Andrew and his mother to confront the father because they were anxious that he would stay away or withdraw even more. Eventually, though, each member of the family was able to say how much his absences cost them and to express their need for his care and involvement. In this case, the parents sought out couples therapy for a period.

In addition to working with Andrew and his family, I spent some time talking with Andrew's schoolteachers. The need for the school to be aware that Andrew was in treatment was important in this case because his symptoms had already resulted in difficulties in his academic and social performance. My goal was to help his teachers appreciate his current difficulties and to help monitor his progress in the classroom without my going into the specifics of Andrew's problems.

As Andrew and his family worked on the relationship between the family's problems and resources and Andrew's behaviors, he began to improve in all aspects. He was less despondent, he become less needy, and he was less regressed, which allowed him to make friends at school.

The key elements in working with a younger school-age child with depressive illness are (1) to relate the therapeutic work to the developmental tasks of the period, especially those of group identification and wishes for mastery; (2) to involve the family in identifying the difficulties with and the solutions to meeting the school-age child's needs; and (3) to include any other relevant institutions in treatment planning, intervention, and monitoring.

The depressed younger school-age child is at risk for difficulties when she enters puberty, a period when her depression may lead to increasingly hazardous behaviors.

Older School-Age Children (Nine- to Twelve-Year-Olds)

In later childhood and the early stages of puberty, children can be particularly vulnerable to depression, especially girls. When working with a child in the early stages of puberty, self-esteem issues are often associated with the physical changes of this period. With girls, concerns about weight and attractiveness are predominant. Boys focus on body size, comparisons with male peers' athletic prowess, and increasing competition in all spheres.

I find this early phase particularly challenging. Kids this age can be as needy and concrete as younger school-age children or as aggressive and sexual as young adults. Their lability is uncomfortable to them and adds to their sense of not feeling much in control. When a depression complicates this picture, these predictable developmental struggles are heightened. Many children in this age group express their depressed symptoms through worry about and disparagement of the physical changes associated with puberty. One depressed boy was so relieved to learn that he could expect to grow another three to four inches in the following years that he was then able to stay in therapy long enough to work on why this was so important to him. Another young girl felt that she was too tall and therefore unattractive. She used the information that she was unlikely to grow much taller as a starting point for exploring other deeper issues of her feelings of diminished self-worth.

With older school-age children, the work is often to build a treatment alliance, as we will see in the next case example. Once this alliance is established, things usually go smoothly, because these children are more verbal and are better self-observers than younger school-age children.

MARGIE

Margie's mother had died two years before Margie, eleven, had begun to experience decreased mood, irritability, decreased school performance, sleep problems, and weight loss. Margie came to my office only after her father insisted. She was difficult to engage. I was finally able to get somewhere when I asked her to use her considerable skill as an artist to draw pictures of her family members. While doing this she was able to discuss her family members and her relationship to them more openly. This strategy worked, because the concrete activity of drawing helped Margie organize some of her feelings. I used this strategy again when we did a similar drawing of

Margie's room and its contents. In this way, she slowly let me into her world and the problems it contained.

After Margie began to trust me, she required fewer of the "structural" aids I used at the beginning, except when she was beginning to explore a difficult topic. When we were able to discuss her mother's death, she required that I return to a more structured kind of support. In this case, I encouraged her simply to describe the events of the funeral and of the days immediately following, without asking that she describe or explore her feelings at first. Once the structure of the events was in place, Margie was able to take on her feelings with more comfort.

In later childhood, most children are still deeply involved in their families and only beginning to experience any ambivalence about them. So with these children I involve the family early and keep them involved during the treatment more than I do with teenagers.

Because her family had suffered a severe loss, Margie was protective of them, and bristled at any suggestion that they played a role in her depression. She was therefore unwilling at first to have them come in for therapy. She ultimately agreed to have a family session, but only because the structure of the meeting would consist of a game.

I asked the family to plan an all-day picnic outing together that included input from all members. After the family did the planning they went on the outing. Predictably, this did not go well, so we were able to identify difficulties in how the family solved problems. They described that there was a disagreement about where to go, which was resolved by the father without discussion. Responsibilities for food and activity planning were handled just as poorly. Instead of a balanced lunch, they had chips, drinks, and cookies. They had planned on playing miniature golf, but found upon arriving that the course was closed. No one had checked to see if the facility was still in operation.

Using this event, we were able to identify specific problems with decision making and management of conflicts and differences in the family. This approach allowed us to work together on the problem-solving difficulties the family was experiencing; I would later apply this understanding to the more sensitive issues about grief and loss that Margie's family was avoiding.

Activities of this sort matched the developmental and emotional limitations of this developmental period. This strategy allowed Margie to protect her family, because the issue of her mother's death and Margie's depression would not be dealt with directly until she and her family were more ready to do so.

Sometimes family therapy is not supported by managed care providers. In Margie's case, the case manager was not experienced in working with school-age children and refused to certify family treatment. She agreed that Margie had a problem, but she could not understand how treating Margie's family would help. Although I tried to educate her on the role of families in children's mental health, she wouldn't change her position. This meant that I needed to appeal the case to their reviewer. In this instance, the reviewer was trained in child development and overruled the decision. The point here is, don't give up if you are initially denied certification. There are always appeal processes, and you should use them in order to secure the best treatment for your patients.

The key elements of working with older school-age children who are moving toward adolescence are (1) to build a rapport based on sharing supportive information about the realities of puberty, (2) to use a strategy to engage the child that recognizes both her cognitive strengths as well as the limitations in this age group, and (3) to involve the family in your work.

SPECIAL PROBLEMS

Some childhood depressions have particular problems associated with them. I discuss those associated with medical illness and sexual abuse in this section because they are two of the most important. My overall approach is the same as with any depressed school-age child, but the circumstances of these children require that I tailor my treatments to meet these special needs.

Medical Illness and Depression

Physical illnesses in childhood have an impact on mental health and are related to increased risk of depression in particular. The degree of depression can be related to a set of risk factors, including the following:

- Illness with early childhood onset (before five years of age) or onset in early adolescence
- Illness that is a result of some environmental exposure (trauma or infection)
- Familial genetics (for example, hemophilia) that may increase feelings of parental guilt and responsibility
- Diagnostic or treatment difficulties
- Illness that causes physical deformity and disability
- Illness with a poor prognosis

For the physically ill child, the most significant problems he experiences in later childhood are governed in large measure by the impact that his illness or its treatment has on his pubertal development. These effects might include influences on the timing of puberty and associated secondary sex characteristics, on body size, or on the development of dysmorphic physical features.

There are many medical illnesses that affect the timing of puberty. The endocrinopathies (for example, Turner's syndrome, a disorder that causes girls not to develop usual female secondary sex characteristics) and genetic anomalies (for example, intersex conditions, in which children are born with ambiguous genitalia) are two examples.

Medical treatments of a variety of illnesses can also affect the timing of puberty. When steroids are used to treat children with chronic and severe asthmatic conditions, for example, secondary sex characteristics may be affected. A secondary effect of changing the timing of puberty is the impact this may have on height and weight.

Specific illnesses and medical treatments may also affect height and weight. For girls, illnesses or treatments that cause weight gain or facial changes are particularly troubling during this phase. For boys, especially at this phase, body size is a significant source of sexual and gender role anxiety. Illnesses that make boys shorter or thinner have a powerfully negative impact on their developing image of themselves as sexual and male. The following case illustrates this problem.

BRAD

Brad was a boy with cystic fibrosis who became depressed and was referred to me by his pulmonologist. Brad weighed a lot less than his peers, which caused a delay in the onset of puberty. Compared to boys his own age, Brad was shorter and more physically immature, which made him the target of harassment from male peers. His struggle with the medical problems of cystic fibrosis was difficult enough, but the social consequences were also devastating. He began to stay away from school, and he became increasingly isolated even from peers who might have been more supportive. He was ashamed of his body and avoided any consideration of sexual thoughts or behaviors. His physician began to be concerned when Brad was repeatedly hospitalized for problems associated with poor compliance with his medical regimen. He was evaluated by a consultation-liaison psychiatrist who recognized the developmental problems Brad was experiencing. We developed supportive and educational therapeutic interventions to assist Brad with his worries about the physical changes associated with the onset of adolescence, and his medical compliance improved, leading to fewer hospitalizations and better psychosexual functioning.

Sexual Abuse and Depression

The subject of sexual abuse and its treatment is covered in Chapter Seven. However, some specific discussion of the impact of sexual abuse on depression is warranted here.

As with any abuse, sexual abuse is likely to have the most severe effects on persons who are young or otherwise vulnerable, when the abuser is a close relative, and when the abuse is violent and ongoing. Shame is a result of sexual abuse that can complicate later psychological functioning and can lead to depression. Shame may result in feelings of being unlovable, feeling damaged and worthless, and feeling different from peers because of this sexual experience. Assisting a child or adolescent with sexual shame requires addressing fundamental ideas of the self and how it has been damaged from abuse. Psychotherapeutic exploration of these issues is currently best formulated in the work of clinicians who use techniques of empathy, mirroring, and other reflecting tools. The following is an example of how sexual abuse affects the onset and treatment of depression.

C . J .

C.J. was a ten-year-old boy who had been sexually abused by his father and uncle and had also been used by them to "recruit" other boys into abuse. He was admitted to the hospital where I worked after he had threatened to commit suicide. C.J. reported depressed mood, problems with sleep and appetite, and persistent and strong impulses to molest a male peer in the group home where he lived. He said the only way to escape these feelings was to die.

C.J. reported that these wishes to molest started getting strong when a female counselor announced she was leaving for a few weeks to get married. C.J. had a strong attachment to the staff member and felt that she was abandoning him. He was so angry with her that he could not speak or look at her.

I understood C.J.'s depression and increased urges to molest as related to the anger and abandonment he felt toward his mother, who allowed C.J.'s father to molest him. Molesting another boy at times seemed preferable to C.J. to feeling powerless and unloved. At the same time, however, he understood how it felt to be the victim of sexual abuse, so he decided that suicide was the only option.

Work with C.J. on these issues required developing a trusting relationship with him and then helping him work on the specific trigger for his current depression. Individual sessions with him focused on his past molestation and his struggles around power. Sessions with the group home staff, including the female counselor, focused on his anxieties about abandonment and feelings of being unlovable and worthless. Initially, this required that I speak for him as he whispered his thoughts in my ear. He would hold his hands over his ears to muffle the female counselor's voice. Eventually he was able to speak and listen without this protection.

After his suicidal wishes diminished and he understood better the origins of his impulses to molest, C.J. returned to the group home. Although he was still recovering from both his sexual abuse and his depression, he was able to continue this work as an outpatient.

Depressed children often endure unfortunate circumstances and sometimes truly heartbreaking events, but my work with such children is some of the most fulfilling work I do. I take special pleasure in play therapy. What I enjoy most about it is figuring out what's "really" going on with a child in the symbolic action of play. Through play, I gain special access to the interior world of the child. With a depressed child, play therapy is an opportunity for the child to experience some relief, and it also allows me to glimpse for short intervals what might be possible for the child to achieve when she recovers.

I also enjoy working with families of school-age children. Although they are often "stressed out" with the work of raising young families and balancing careers, they make good family therapy cases because everyone can talk to one another. The children are neither too young to fully participate nor are they involved in an adolescent struggle to get out of the family. Because school-age children are less conflicted about their parents than are adolescents, they are often better allies in the process of family therapy.

I am usually hopeful when I begin treating a school-age child with depression. Although I am aware that children with depression in their school-age years are more likely to experience future depressions, I believe that we now have a better understanding of how to help those who are lucky enough to be identified.

NOTES

P. 66, *Studies of seriously deprived infants:* Spitz, R. (1945). Hospitalism: An inquiry into the genesis of psychiatric conditions in early childhood. *Psychoanalytic Study of the Child, 1,* p. 53.

P. 66, *About 2 percent of these school-age children:* Kashani, J. H., & Sherman, D. D. (1988). Childhood depression: Epidemiology, etiological models, and treatment implications. *Integrative Psychiatry, 6,* 1–8.

P. 66, *studies of pediatric medical patients:* Kashani, J. H., Barbera, G. H., & Bolander, F. D., (1981). Depression in hospitalized pediatric patients. *Journal of the Academy of Child and Adolescent Psychiatry, 20,* 123–134.

P. 67, *If there is a family history of depression:* Warner, V., Mufson, J., & Weissman, M. (1995). Offspring at high- and low-risk for depression and anxiety: Mechanisms of psychiatric disorder. *Journal of the American Academy of Child and Adolescent Psychiatry, 34*(6), 786–797.

P. 69, *to be diagnosed with Major Depression:* American Psychiatric Association. (1994). *Diagnostic and statistical manual of mental disorders* (4th ed.). Washington, DC: Author, p. 327.

P. 70, *The* DSM-IV *describes Dysthymia:* American Psychiatric Association. (1994). *ibid.*, p. 349.

P. 72, *The* DSM-IV *requires that the person experiences hypomania:* American Psychiatric Association. (1994). *ibid.*, p. 365.

P. 75, *Only recently have carefully conducted studies:* Ambrosini, R., Bianchi, M., Rabinovich, J., & Elia, J. (1993). Antidepressant treatments in children and adolescents: Vol. I. Affective disorders. *Journal of the American Academy of Child and Adolescent Psychiatry, 32,* 1–6.

P. 87, *The degree of depression can be related to a set of risk factors:* Mrazak, D. (1991). Chronic pediatric illness and multiple hospitalizations. In M. Lewis (Ed.), *Child and adolescent psychiatry: A comprehensive textbook.* Baltimore: Williams & Wilkins, p. 1049.

4

DISRUPTIVE BEHAVIORAL DISORDERS

Lisa R. Benton-Hardy and James Lock

Disruptive behavioral disorders are a common problem for children, especially when they are in school. These behaviors can be challenging to differentiate from normal behavior and very difficult to treat. Diagnosis is difficult because at times almost all children misbehave and have trouble following rules. Treatment is also challenging: disruptive behaviors are more a problem to other people—parents and teachers—than to the child, so it's often hard to enlist the child's cooperation with evaluation and treatment. However, because of their potential negative impact on school functioning, peer and family relationships, and long-term functioning, the behaviors are important to identify and manage. In our capacity as clinicians at a university medical center, we are frequently called upon to evaluate children with disruptive behaviors. This chapter represents our particular approach to evaluation and treatment, which is based on years of experience with these disorders.

In this chapter we review the following disorders: Attention Deficit Hyperactivity Disorder, Oppositional Defiant Disorder, and Conduct Disorder. Because Conduct Disorder is much less common in school-age children, we review it only briefly. (For more information about this disorder, please see *Treating Adolescents*, another volume in this series.)

ATTENTION DEFICIT
HYPERACTIVITY DISORDER: DIAGNOSIS

Attention Deficit Hyperactivity Disorder (ADHD) has become one of the most widely used and some say abused diagnoses today. Although the reasons for its popularity are unclear, one possible reason is that it provides a way to understand and manage many of the more troublesome behaviors of children and to explain why some do poorly in school. Because about a third of the children diagnosed with ADHD will continue to have symptoms beyond childhood, it is important to begin diagnosing and treating them as soon as possible. Also, untreated ADHD can cause problems with school and with forming relationships, thus significantly affecting long-term adjustment and achievements.

ADAM

Adam's mother said that he was overactive in the womb. He walked early and was a "climber." He was curious and constantly into things from an early age. His mother reported that by the time Adam was age three, she spent her days chasing after him and struggling with his many mishaps. When Adam was four his mother started back to work, and he started preschool. Adam's mother continued to hope that the structure of school and having other boys to play with would "run it out of him." In fact, the opposite was the case: Adam's behavior worsened in the structured preschool program. His mother was called almost every day because Adam wouldn't or couldn't follow simple routines and had increasing difficulty playing with his peers. Sometimes he hit other children, and they began to avoid him. Adam's mother changed preschools; the new one was less structured and used more physical activity, and Adam did somewhat better.

When Adam started kindergarten, his teachers noted that he was inattentive and couldn't sit still for even a short period. He continued to have difficulty with peers. He performed poorly in first grade; his teacher suspected that he had a learning disability and suggested Adam be referred to a psychiatrist for evaluation.

Adam came into the office with his mother and sat in a chair. He had a cut on his knee and a yellowing bruise on his arm. He sat quietly in his chair for a few minutes as his mother related his story. After a few minutes, Adam had difficulty sitting still and began to fidget. Soon he turned around and began to play with the magazines on the table beside him. He interrupted his mother to ask for a candy he had been promised if he behaved well during the interview.

In the playroom, Adam displayed great energy and interest. He opened all the toy cabinets and pulled out toy after toy, hardly stopping long enough to look at them, let alone play with them. He began to throw a ball around the room, and he tipped over a small lamp. Although he was friendly and interested enough in talking, he was clearly unable to stop long enough to focus on what was being asked. We concluded the interview when Adam's enthusiasm for the toys diminished, and he left the playroom calling loudly for his mother as he ran down the hall.

Symptoms and Causes

The key features of ADHD include difficulty paying attention, restlessness or difficulty sitting still, and impulsivity. These features must be present before age seven and cause significant problems at home and at school and often in other settings. As you can imagine, a child with these characteristics may have trouble paying attention to what parents, teachers, and friends say; following rules and obeying limits; and getting along with others. ADHD is thought to describe 2 to 6 percent of children. It seems to affect boys more than girls at a rate of four to one.

Girls often present with more subtle signs of ADHD; they may be less restless and less impulsive. Consequently, a thorough evaluation is particularly important when evaluating girls. You need to pay special attention to problems with inattention, inability to perform up to expected academic capacities, and general disorganization. Because these problems affect mostly the child herself, teachers and parents don't always "notice" girls having problems with inattention and distractibility and often assume these behaviors are due to being unintelligent. This may be responsible for the higher reported rate of ADHD in boys; because their behaviors are more disruptive and apparent, boys may be referred for evaluation more frequently. In the developing diagnostic nomenclature of the *DSM*, girls are more often correctly diagnosed as having attention deficit disorder without hyperactivity.

Although the cause of ADHD is not clear, it seems likely that this problem stems from a combination of genetic and environmental factors. Children of parents with ADHD seem to be twice as likely to develop ADHD. Structural and neurochemical differences in the brains of children with ADHD have also been suggested. Potential environmental factors include exposures to toxins (such as lead) and the influence of certain parenting styles. Family stress and a poor mother-child relationship are frequently found among children with ADHD. Inconsistent parenting and limited financial and social resources are also implicated. We propose that the primary basis is a genetic and neuroanatomical predisposition, which is then mitigated or exacerbated by the familial and social environment.

Assessment

In order to decide if a child has ADHD, we find it helpful to interview the child, the family, schoolteachers, and anyone else who may have had a chance to observe the behaviors in question. Often, different people observe and complain of different things, so it is extremely useful to get everyone's perspective before making a diagnosis and initiating treatment. This is not only because people have different points of view but because the behaviors themselves may change in different settings and under different conditions. Often a child may appear quiet and subdued in the playroom but become easily disruptive and restless at school.

Our assessment of the child also focuses on a direct observation of his behavior, style of play, and ability to interact during the play session. If a child has enrolled in school or seems more able to express himself verbally, we will often ask the child if there are situations that just don't seem to be going well. Does he find it hard to sit still in class? Does he find himself frequently daydreaming and having difficulty listening to the teacher? Are homework assignments hard to complete or understand? Is he able to play and get along well with other kids? Some children, despite their age, are amazingly able to share their experiences and can often be an overlooked source of valuable information.

Next we interview the parents to review birth and developmental history (especially any history of trauma), beginning of symptoms, times and settings when symptoms occur, and things that exacerbate or ameliorate symptoms. We also ask about family history of ADHD, other psychiatric problems, and other nonpsychiatric medical problems. We try to get a picture of what the family environment is like and how the family members have coped with and managed the problematic behaviors. We ask the parents to be as specific as possible and encourage them to continue the dialog with teachers and other significant adults. This is particularly important to emphasize, as the entry into school often exacerbates the behaviors and brings them to parents' and others' attention in different ways than before. The increased need for concentration, self-direction, and compliance with rules makes the behaviors particularly apparent. Educational testing is also a useful means of evaluating the child for the presence of learning disorders, which can mimic and complicate ADHD. Educational testing allows us to begin thinking about what additional tests we may need, such as neurological screening. Additionally, it provides a more objective assessment of the child.

In evaluating a child for ADHD, we remain aware of other syndromes that can mimic ADHD. The child who has separation anxiety or a phobia may appear restless, agitated, and disobedient when faced with going to school or leaving the parents' side. A child who is depressed may have trouble concentrating, seem easily distracted, and have trouble completing projects or assignments. A report of restlessness and distractibility when other children are sitting quietly is a helpful clue. Situations with multiple stimuli also seem to bring out ADHD symptoms, as the child becomes overwhelmed and their fragile organizing structure dissolves.

Additional concerns to keep in mind include the concurrent presence of Oppositional Defiant Disorder (ODD) or possibly Conduct Disorder (CD). Up to 40 percent of children with ADHD can develop ODD and later CD (this latter condition is unusual in children under the age of ten). When we interview children for ADHD, we anticipate that a child is likely to meet criteria for another diagnosis and plan for this possibility. This may mean additional medication, psychotherapy, and family support. This more intensive treatment is important because the prognosis is poorer when children have an additional diagnosis, especially if it is a behavioral disorder.

In Adam's case, our trip to the playroom was an assessment opportunity. By letting Adam decide how he would "play" we were able to see the degree of difficulty he had organizing himself, choosing a toy, paying attention to what he was doing, and even enjoying the toys at all. In addition, we could see the chaos, havoc, mess, and potential for injury that attended Adam's inattention and distractibility. It was also easy to see how accidents could be perceived to be aggressive actions, considering that much of the stimulation of throwing things was unfocused and undirected. Adam's playroom behavior is classic for a boy with hyperactivity and inattention problems.

However, a single trip to a playroom is not sufficient for evaluation, so we use one of the variety of instruments available to aid in the diagnosis of ADHD. These can be used by parents and teachers as well as therapists. The most common is the Conners Behavioral Checklist. It provides a list of behaviors that allows the rater to define the breadth and depth of problematic behaviors. Although we do not suggest using this instrument in place of a good clinical assessment, it can provide additional validation of the diagnosis if the scores are high enough. It also can provide an objective way of monitoring the progress of children throughout treatment.

Observing the child at school, if you are able to do so, can be very informative. The structure of the classroom almost always adds to the difficulty that these children have in organizing their activities. Although this idea may seem counterintuitive, it makes sense if you think of ADHD as an illness that causes a child to seek constant stimulation; any diminishment of stimulation—whether caused by sitting or by focusing on just one thing—leads to difficulties. In a classroom, you will see how the child with ADHD becomes the target of jokes because of a seeming inability and disregard for the group behavioral norms. You will also see how inattention and distraction make learning impossible and can lead to children with ADHD becoming oppositional in order to be relieved of the embarrassment of being unable to attend and conform.

Family evaluations are also important, because the family has had to cope with the chronic difficulties associated with living with a child with ADHD. Typically, the child feels constantly criticized and harassed, and harbors feelings of anger and resentment. On the other hand, the other family members are also irritated and frustrated with their inability to control the constant activity, accidents, and disobedience that result from the child's inattention and overactivity. Parents complain that their child with ADHD never completes anything, that they find the stove on or the refrigerator open and a trail of belongings following the child. Siblings complain of being hit, ignored, and frustrated. Often, the astute clinician will see evidence of at least one other family member with ADHD.

ADHD: Pharmacological and Psychotherapeutic Treatments

The two major approaches to treating ADHD are pharmacological and psychotherapeutic treatments. In recent years, we have advanced our understanding of the role of medications in treating ADHD, and the number and types of medication available have increased. This is a great advance, but we have also learned that medication alone is seldom sufficient as an approach to treating children with ADHD. Instead, a multimodal approach is best—one that incorporates both medication and psychotherapeutic interventions.

Medications

Among the variety of treatments available, medications are often effective. The most common medications used to treat ADHD are the psychostimulants: methylphenidate (Ritalin) and dextroamphetamine (Dexedrine). This group of medications is effective in most children (up to 75 percent) and helps with motor control, attention, short-term memory, impulsivity, aggression, and oppositionality. Newer medications are also currently being evaluated for treatment of ADHD, including clonidine, Prozac, and other antidepressants. None of these medications have been found to be superior to the psychostimulants in treating the symptoms of ADHD, but some children tolerate them better.

When working with medication, it is important to develop an alliance with the parents. We review both the potential benefits and the risks of medication and also establish target symptoms to provide a means of assessing the ongoing need for and usefulness of medication. Following target symptoms is particularly important, and we like to do this at each medication visit, verbally and in writing. Although we are candid about risks, we emphasize the established safety of the medicine and our commitment to work with the parents and child and to continually reassess the need for medication. When used properly, Ritalin and the other psychostimulants are very effective and can produce dramatic changes in a child's behavior.

Many parents are justifiably concerned about long-term risks and potential effects on growth and development. However, these risks can be minimized with proper management. Other risks include the development of motor and tic disorders, appetite suppression, some stomach discomfort, difficulty sleeping, and cognitive dulling or confusion. Informing parents of the potential side effects usually doesn't turn them off to using medication; rather, we find that it often makes medication management go more smoothly, because parents can alert us to problems. In Adam's case, his mother was reluctant to try medication at first. However, we did convince her to try it for a short period so that she would be able to see for herself if Adam responded. Luckily, he did, and he had no complications with moderate doses.

Because of the usefulness of medication treatment and its ability to facilitate other forms of treatment, we spend a great deal of time making sure things are clear and understood. If medication is the only aspect of treatment that we are involved in, we find it crucial to communicate regularly with the other people involved. Of course, you must also keep in mind that even though they are effective, medications are not "magic pills" that cure everything. There is still an important place for behavioral programs and individual and family therapy.

Individual Therapy

The main role of individual therapy is to help the child learn to manage some of the impulses and aggressions he has and to provide a chance to explore how the ADHD is affecting the child's self-esteem and relationships with others. To this end, we have used a combination of supportive (strengthening the child's adaptive structure) and expressive (gently challenging and exploring possible beneficial changes in the adaptive structure) psychotherapy. Children with ADHD often function at a level younger than their chronological age. This is helpful to keep in mind when choosing activities for play therapy and when evaluating the child's ability to do certain activities.

Adam had had long-standing problems that interfered with his family, peer, and school performance. As a result, when we started therapy he was quite negative and expressed this by making many critical comments about himself, such as, "Oh, I did it again, I'm really bad at writing. Look how awful the picture I drew is." He was reluctant to see much of value in anything he could do, and it required substantial effort to identify some of his strengths. Even after he had some response to Ritalin and was more able to focus and perform, his expectations of himself were low. In our work together, we employed a strategy of storytelling that permitted him to externalize some of his negative feelings. This technique also allowed us to interact and comment on the behaviors of fantasy figures, protecting the child from the confrontational aspect of interpretations to a certain degree. Adam described a boy named Mike who was no good at anything and who decided to run away. This allowed an interpretation of how angry and sad Mike must be to want to run away. Adam said that this was true for Mike and that sometimes he felt this way too. Over time, supportive, gentle exploratory work of this kind can help to ameliorate the long-term pain that having ADHD has generated in the child.

Family Therapy

As in individual therapy, there is a role in family therapy for both supportive and expressive psychotherapy. Acting as a resource for the family and helping them learn ways to manage the child's behavior are the main focuses for family therapy. Often parents are exhausted from trying to control their child's behavior. Reassuring them that this is normal and does not make them bad parents is important. In addition to these educational and supportive therapeutic techniques, it is also important to explore how the child with ADHD has affected family functioning over time. This history often plays a significant role in perpetuating behavioral and emotional problems in the child that are not directly related to the symptoms of ADHD.

Cognitive approaches to these problems can help a family identify ways the child's behavior has changed and to recognize and reward the child for making these changes. Emotional expression of past anger and frustration on the part of family members can help clear the road for future changes. It is also important that the child express how she felt to be criticized and punished for things that she felt were beyond her control.

Work with Adam's family proceeded much along these lines. Psychoeducation in the early sessions helped all family members appreciate the problems Adam was having in conforming to their expectations. Next, the family spent several sessions identifying progress that Adam was making. This supported the changes in Adam's behavior and provided a new emotional frame for him, one that he experienced as less critical and more understanding of his difficulties. With this improved family milieu it was safe for Adam and his family to express the more difficult feelings of anger and frustration that had been such a big part of the family's emotional life prior to Adam's treatment.

Group Therapy

Some children can benefit from small-group support for the development of age-appropriate social and relationship skills in the context of treatment for ADHD. Small groups of children with ADHD can benefit from structured approaches to learning to cooperate, share, accomplish tasks, and make friends. Such groups often use a reward system (such as a star chart or a point system) for specific behavioral accomplishments. In addition, a plan with progressive difficulty within age-appropriate norms makes group work appealing for the child. For example, a starting activity might be to build a model, then later to build a model with a single peer. The aim of such groups is to assist children with ADHD to catch up with their peers in some of the social skills areas that are affected as a consequence of ADHD. We treated five boys, ages eight to ten, using a group approach. Over the one-year course of treatment, the boys were able to increase their cooperative skills and decrease their aggression. Their progress is best illustrated by the increasing complexity of their cooperative achievements: at first they couldn't even sit at a table together for more than a few minutes, but by the end of the first three months, they were able to plan, draw, and paint a holiday mural together. At the end of a year of group treatment, they wrote a story, illustrated it, and copied and bound it together for their families.

School Consultation

Another important part of treatment is continuing contact with the child's school and involved teacher. By including the teacher in the treatment plan, you gain an important ally. Just as teachers are often the first to call attention to the problem behaviors, they are also in an excellent position to monitor the effects of the treatment. Frequent contact with the school and the teacher is essential. Often, modifications may need to be made in the classroom as well as at home to better control the behaviors. Examples include more individual teaching time, more frequent follow-up with parents, and assigning a task in smaller pieces rather than all at once.

Managed Care

Too often these days, limits on health care benefits prohibit full diagnostic procedures and follow-up. Worse still, many mental health insurance plans specifically exclude treatment of ADHD. Considering that ADHD is one of the most common childhood mental health problems, this exclusion can be a major barrier. Unfortunately, it has become common practice to "disguise" the diagnosis of ADHD by calling it something else—such as depression or anxiety. Although it may be expeditious to do so, it often mislabels a child and may lead to problems with coverage down the road.

Under many managed care plans, pediatricians are the gatekeepers. They are often the first to diagnose and treat ADHD (at least with medications). Unfortunately, many pediatricians haven't the time or expertise to make this diagnosis and do not keep up with newer methods of treatment. Sometimes the best approach to this kind of problem is for you to develop a consultative relationship with a pediatrician. That way, initial evaluations and treatment plans are more likely to be appropriate.

When there is coverage for ADHD in the mental health insurance policy, it still is often necessary to educate case managers about what helps kids with ADHD. There is a strong bias toward medication use in such plans because it appears to be quicker and cheaper. Case managers need to be told about all features of the illness—the familial and social-behavioral dimensions particularly—so that they understand the need for the multimodal kind of treatment we think is most effective. We have found that discussing the need to prevent future emotional, occupational, and familial problems helps us get certification for treatments that are needed.

Outcomes

Children with ADHD generally fall into three outcome groups. About 20 percent continue to have trouble into adolescence but function fairly well in adulthood. The vast majority fall into a second group, who continue to have difficulties with attention, concentration, impulsiveness, and social and emotional functioning, but these problems are generally manageable with ongoing support. A relatively small minority of children grow up to have significant psychopathology associated with serious depression and to exhibit antisocial behaviors. Children appear to be more likely to fall into this third group if there are family members with mental health problems, lower IQ, or lower socioeconomic status. In addition, when severe problems with aggression and conduct exist together with ADHD, poorer outcomes are expected.

ADHD is one of the most common and, happily, one of the most treatable childhood behavior disorders. Dealing with the difficulties of making the correct diagnosis and of organizing the child and his family for effective treatment is the real trick. The strategies described here should help get you started on the right track in both these regards. Because ADHD starts off as a limited syndrome of problems with attention, distractibility, and overactivity, but can end in problems that extend into all domains of a child's life, it is important that you accurately diagnose and adequately treat ADHD. Medication clearly is not a panacea, and even when it is used, it must be used in the context of an overall treatment plan. Pediatricians and some psychiatrists have tried to avoid addressing the whole child in their treatment of ADHD, but they find that their outcomes are far from satisfying. Medication noncompliance, increased behavioral problems, and finally conduct and perhaps substance abuse problems may develop that might have been prevented.

OPPOSITIONAL DEFIANT DISORDER: DIAGNOSIS

ANTHONY

Anthony, age seven, was sent to us for an urgent psychiatric evaluation because the medical team was having more and more trouble treating his leukemia. When he would come for his appointments he would not allow members of the team to examine him, let alone administer his treatments or get lab draws. If someone did try he would scream, curse, and often assault the person with punches and bites. On one particular visit, he began swinging a pole around his head to stop a lab draw and seriously injured someone. During these outbursts, his mother was powerless to control him and often became injured herself. She would initially try to manage his behavior by talking to him calmly, and failing that would try to restrain him physically. As this was also ineffective, she would eventually give up, and she often began crying from disappointment and embarrassment with his behavior.

At home, the situation was not much better. His mother reported that Anthony "ran the household." He refused to do any of his chores or homework, and when asked to do something he did not want to do he would throw a tantrum and attack anyone within range. At school, he was often sent to the corner for time-outs after disrupting class and was unwilling to complete any of his assignments or follow any of the instructions the teacher gave him. In all respects, the situation was becoming increasingly more difficult for everyone involved in his care, and the family felt "at the end of their rope."

Anthony's problems are typical of Oppositional Defiant Disorder (ODD). The continued problem of disobedient, defiant, and occasionally hostile behavior, usually directed toward an authority figure, is described in the *DSM-IV* as the central feature of the disorder. The behaviors must have been present for at least six months and must include at least four of the following:

- Often loses temper
- Often argues with adults
- Defies authority
- Often intentionally annoys people
- Blames others for his own misbehavior and mistakes
- Easily annoyed and irritated by others
- Frequently angry
- Frequently spiteful or vindictive

Additionally, given the overlap between these behaviors and those seen with mood and psychotic disorders, the behaviors can't occur as part of a mood or psychotic disorder and must cause clinically significant impairment in family, school, or social functioning.

After Conduct Disorder, which we discuss in the next section, ODD represents the second most frequent behavior problem associated with psychiatric referral in school-age children. It is considered to be a relatively common disorder of childhood; the prevalence is estimated to be 1.5 to 10 percent of the general population. It is two to three times more common among school-age boys than girls. Most children begin with problems in early childhood, and cases seldom start after age ten. The precise etiology of ODD is unknown. Currently we believe that it is multifactorial and stems from a combination of genetic and environmental factors. Environmental factors include family and marital discord; family history of disruptive behavioral disorders, mood disorders, or substance abuse; and parenting styles characterized by unavailability, inconsistent discipline, or permissiveness. Additionally, the interaction between the parent's style of parenting and the child's temperament is likely to affect the development of oppositional behavior.

Because the oppositional behavior may represent a normal phase of early childhood development, diagnosing ODD is particularly difficult. Information about a child's developmental history is important. Were there early conflicts and difficulties following parental instructions? The child's reaction to toilet training, early chores, and outside obligations (such as homework or school assignments) can be quite telling. The degree of argumentativeness and hostility is usually beyond that expected of the particular situation. Serious problems—stealing, lying, and overt cruelty and harm to others—are not typically present, and if they are, they may be a precursor of a later diagnosis of Conduct Disorder.

The initial differential diagnosis for ODD includes the other disruptive behavioral disorders, ADHD and Conduct Disorder.

Although many children with ODD may have impulsivity and hyperactivity as presenting problems, most lack attentional deficits. In fact, many can be amazingly focused and tenacious in the midst of a conflict or argument. Also, because of the behaviors, ODD tends to be more disruptive of family and peer relationships. The distinction between ODD and Conduct Disorder is more difficult; many have considered ODD to be a milder form or precursor of Conduct Disorder. However, most children with ODD lack the key features of Conduct Disorder (disregard for the rights of others and overt cruelty to others). One caveat is in order, though. In many children with ODD, the decision is not whether the child has either ODD or ADHD or Conduct Disorder but whether the child has both ODD and ADHD or ODD and Conduct Disorder. Studies have shown that 33 percent of children may have two concurrent behavior disorders, and 2 percent may actually have all three! The association between ODD and ADHD is particularly strong. Thus, in these children, diagnosis becomes a complicated issue. Other co-morbid conditions in school-age children include anxiety disorders and learning disorders. In older children, substance abuse and mood disorders may further cloud the picture. Accurate diagnosis depends on a careful assessment of the child, the family, and the child's behavior in multiple settings.

ODD: PHARMACOLOGICAL AND PSYCHOTHERAPEUTIC TREATMENTS

Treating ODD can be a big challenge. However, once the behaviors are under control, it can be truly amazing to see how these children's lives can turn around. Many begin to do well at school and at home and form more appropriate and warm peer relations. Approach to the treatment of ODD usually entails the use of many different treatment modalities. Generally the emphasis is on psychotherapy and behavior modification rather than on medication.

Treatment Setting

The first question to answer relates to the setting of treatment. This is usually determined by the child himself. If the behaviors are severe and pose a danger to others or to the child, hospitalization can be a valuable intervention. If the family situation is chaotic and if family members are unavailable or inaccessible, the ability to house a child within a structured, calm setting can be invaluable. This allows for a more thorough assessment of both the child and the family. Use pharmacological treatment as needed. Firm but supportive behavioral programs are essential. After the child has been stabilized, the goal is to return him to the home environment as soon as possible. Transitioning to outpatient treatment allows more definitive, long-term treatment to start while all are still actively committed and involved. In today's managed care environment, it is often difficult to hospitalize a child with ODD. It is mandatory that you discuss with case managers the need for a safe environment for evaluation when a child's behavior is out of control. Subacute or day treatment settings, if available, might be viable options for initial evaluation or for early transition out of hospital care.

Medications

With both inpatients and outpatients, an important aspect of treatment involves the early identification of co-morbid conditions. If a child has an anxiety or mood disorder, it is desirable to treat this condition first (especially because more definitive treatment guidelines are available) and then reassess the oppositional behavior. Medication can be helpful and is often started during a hospitalization. Your choice of medication relates to specific target symptoms: psychostimulants and clonidine for the impulsivity and hyperactivity of ADHD, tricyclics and serotonin inhibitors for depression and neurovegetative symptoms, and benadryl for anxiety. Because of the young age of the child, we try to use medications sparingly and only when indicated. In these cases, treating these other conditions may make the oppositional behaviors less problematic and more manageable.

Individual Therapy

Forming an alliance with a child with oppositional behaviors and creating an environment where the role of these behaviors can be explored are not easy tasks. The very reason the child has come to you for treatment is because he is unable to follow directions without angry, hostile (and often harmful) behavior. Sometimes it requires several sessions before the child can even tolerate and participate in therapy. In the meantime, we often find ourselves becoming more angry and impatient, often almost mirroring the child's behaviors! But once therapy becomes accepted, the underlying issues—often insecurity, depression, and powerlessness—unfold and can be worked through quite successfully. Let's return to our case study with Anthony to explore these and other issues of individual therapy with the child with ODD.

The first session with Anthony seemed to be a complete disaster. It required at least fifteen minutes before he was willing to enter the playroom with his mother and explore the toys. During that time he was yelling, cursing, and striking at his mom whenever she tried to lead him into the playroom. After he entered the room, the first thing he did was to overturn a large basket of toys and begin throwing them around the room. When I (Benton-Hardy) tried to establish some limits on his behavior, he began throwing the toys at me and tried to kick me. Eventually, after much cajoling by his mother, he calmed down slightly and began to concentrate his efforts on a toy phone, which he began banging on the floor. He still refused to look at me or play with me; he refused to talk except to curse from time to time. After a short while he again became angry and agitated.

It seemed as though both he and I were in danger of harm, so we ended the session.

As mentioned previously, the issue of safety comes up often with children with ODD. We try to allow the child to play spontaneously and to feel free to explore the room and the toys. However, you may need to set limits regarding what is acceptable behavior and what is not. If either you or the child appears to be in danger because of the nature of the behaviors, we recommend ending the session or taking a break until safety is restored. Many of the children we work with come from families in which effective limits were not set or maintained. Paradoxically, it is often comforting and reassuring to these children when an adult takes the initiative to establish and maintain limits. Clear limits, patience, and tolerance of some negative behavior are imperative.

Other strategies to create a safe, supportive environment include establishing the basic structure of therapy and discussing appropriate rules of therapy at the start. These include starting and finishing on time, letting the child know which areas of the office are off-limits (that is, closed cabinet doors are to stay closed, books on shelves are to stay on shelves, and so forth) and what some of the goals of therapy are (a way for us to get to know each other and to find a way to understand what's going wrong at home and school). Often we find it helpful to play in one area of the room initially with only one or two toys to limit the amount of potential stimulation and distraction. Playing games can be especially valuable, as the games illustrate how the child may be having difficulty following rules. By establishing a framework, tolerating some misbehavior, and adhering to appropriate limits, we try to create a situation in which we can develop rapport and explore the child's difficulties. Meeting initially with the child in the parent's presence can also be beneficial, if the parent is able to settle the child and help redirect his behavior. Help from the parent allows you to concentrate more on being a therapist rather than a policeman. If the parent seems prone to getting into power struggles with the child and revving the child up, however, you may want to consider meeting alone with the child. Your goal is to create an environment to explore the behaviors, not to replicate or feed them.

Paradoxically, some children can be quite charming and engaging at first. In these cases you should proceed with caution and remain aware of the anger that may be lurking beneath the surface. Some of these children have a history of trauma and neglect. Although this does not justify the behaviors, it does provide a means for understanding them. Again, patience, perseverance, and tolerance of negative situations are valuable tools for you to possess. Cognitive behavior therapy may also be helpful. It can enhance a child's sense of self-control and begin providing nonviolent ways to approach problems.

The next two sessions resembled the first. However, at the end of the third session I tried a different approach. During the first two sessions, I had remained a somewhat passive participant: I concentrated on maintaining the framework, making sure no one was hurt, and remaining supportive and nonjudgmental. When Anthony was getting ready to leave, I thanked him for coming to see me and for allowing me to get to know him and to understand what was going on from his point of view. I mentioned that it must have been very hard to play at times and to try to follow the rules I had set about not throwing toys at me or breaking things (an example of an interpretation). He suddenly began to cry and seemed to curl up into a tight little ball. His mother began crying softly as well but made no move to comfort him. I moved closer to him and began rubbing his shoulder. He relaxed somewhat and then said, "I really miss my dad." After five minutes of silence, he stopped crying, shoved me away, and began once again throwing toys at the wall.

The decision to use interpretation in therapy is often a difficult one. Usually, it's best to wait until there is a fairly strong alliance between you and the child and when the validity of the interpretation is pretty clear. However, sometimes interpretations at the beginning of therapy are also useful. If they are appropriate, as in Anthony's case, they can strengthen the alliance and open new areas of exploration.

Using interpretation illustrates another aspect of therapy that we think is very important in working with oppositional children. Children with oppositional behaviors have often received predominantly punishment and rejection because of their behaviors; their strengths may have gone unnoticed. Consequently, we recommend complimenting them on their abilities and avoiding comments on their limitations. Along these lines, we recommend staying out of the power struggle and trying to remain a neutral, although supportive, observer. This can be especially difficult, yet it is a critical element of working with oppositional children. Therapy should remain a safe space for play and exploration, not a place to replicate the problems it is supposed to correct.

Family Therapy

The other mainstay in the treatment of ODD is family therapy. Because most young children spend the majority of their time with their parents (school and the peer group have not become as influential), it is critical to enlist the family's support for individual work and participation in family therapy.

As with the child, this is often hard to do. The very reasons the child may have developed ODD can make it difficult to form an alliance with the family: inconsistency, unavailability, and noncompliance are formidable obstacles to overcome. To foster family support, we begin by providing educational material about the problem behaviors. We also spend some time exploring what parental issues may be contributing to the development and perpetuation of the problem behaviors. Because of their own childhood and developmental experiences, many parents have problems establishing limits and rules for their child's behaviors. Sometimes, even when they do establish a rule, they don't follow through. They fail to reward good behavior or redirect negative behavior.

Meeting with the parents separately to teach parenting skills geared toward reducing the aggressive and antisocial behavior can be helpful. Positively reinforcing prosocial behavior and negatively diminishing antisocial behavior can be very effective yet require a level of dedication and consistency that many of these parents lack. Creating a more structured home environment is also useful. To this end you can recommend guidelines such as (1) establishing house rules (and making clear what the consequences are for disobeying these rules), (2) being consistent with enforcing rules, (3) monitoring a child's behavior and feeling states, and (4) establishing ways to resolve conflicts and disagreements. Although these guidelines generally apply to all families, we believe that families with children who have ODD require a higher level of flexibility, patience, and perseverance.

Managed Care

As we discussed earlier, hospitalization for ODD can be difficult under managed care plans because of the cost of such a setting. Unfortunately, outpatient problems with managed care also can inhibit treatment of children with ODD. Many case managers believe that these are just "bad kids" and that mental health practitioners can do little to help them. Since this is not the case, it falls to you to educate them about what is possible. Usually, it is necessary to develop a comprehensive treatment plan with specific goals and outcomes. Be careful not to make these too grandiose; instead develop a step-by-step plan. For example, start with a plan for a complete individual and family evaluation over three sessions. Next, develop a behavioral plan to address the most significant difficulties. If the behavioral problems involve aggression toward family members or peers, this is a good place to start. Continue to develop and refine these behavioral interventions and goals, and keep up a discussion with the case manager about your progress. This increases the case manager's investment in your success. When the inevitable setbacks arise, be sure to address these with alternative plans. This reassures reviewers that you are continuing to actively pursue treatment goals, and this in turn allows them to justify continued approval of treatment sessions. The overall rule is to be prepared with educational material and reasonable plans whenever you speak to a reviewer.

Outcomes

The prognosis of children with ODD depends a great deal on the timeliness of the intervention and the child and family's response. Mean duration is approximately 4.5 years, although symptoms that started in childhood may continue into adolescence and adulthood in up to 14 percent of cases. If an intervention is successful, many children can get back on track and have improved family, school, and peer relations. If there is no intervention or if treatment is unsuccessful, many of these children can go on to develop Conduct Disorder and possibly Antisocial Personality Disorder, both of which have a poorer prognosis.

CONDUCT DISORDER: DIAGNOSIS AND TREATMENT

MATTHEW

Matthew had been involved in gangs for most of his young life. He grew up with his mother and siblings; his father had died when Matthew was fairly young, and prior to his death had had limited contact with Matthew, as he had been on drugs and in and out of jail. Likewise, Matthew's mother had a history of drug use and prostitution. Despite his parents' unavailability and unreliability, Matthew had learned to develop strong emotional ties to adults. He was close to his maternal grandmother and looked up to his older brother. Unfortunately, as his grandmother was less able to provide clear limits and modeling of important values, he began to imitate his brother. He became involved in gangs by the time he was eight, trying to outdo his brother, who was either in detention or jail most of the time. He had a lengthy history of vandalism, disrupting the peace, theft, robbery, and assault. He began abusing drugs at age ten and was considering selling drugs to prove himself. He was quick to use guns and knives to handle disagreements and only came to the attention of police after a two-day crime spree during which he robbed and shot several people.

Conduct Disorder (CD) is generally recognized as the most common form of late-childhood and teenage behavioral problems. It is a common reason for referral, accounting for 30 to 50 percent of referrals in some clinics. It is found mainly in boys (at a rate of three to one compared to girls), and the general prevalence is estimated to be 2 to 10 percent. The gender difference decreases with adolescence, and because of the difficulty in diagnosing early onset antisocial behavior in girls, the number of girls with CD may actually be higher than reported. This is because girls engage in more covert activities, such as substance abuse, petty theft, and promiscuity, whereas boys participate in more overt behaviors, such as vandalism and assault.

Diagnosis

As was true in Anthony's case, conduct disordered behavior makes you think of the stereotypical juvenile delinquent. The basic feature is a pattern of behavior that violates the rights of others and represents a departure from age-appropriate and societally appropriate behavior. Teenagers will often show such behaviors as aggression to animals and people, property destruction, theft or deceit, and serious violation of rules. Additionally, the behaviors must lead to significant trouble functioning at home or at school.

Although Conduct Disorder is mainly a diagnosis of late childhood to the early teens, many of the behaviors can be shown to have started in early childhood. Such characteristics as stubbornness, being quick tempered, and being easily prone to temper tantrums and angry outbursts are common. Opposition to parents and problems at home are common. More covert behavior may appear as the child is faced with the challenges of school and peers, and some children begin to lie and engage in mild forms of delinquency (vandalism and stealing). Eventually these behaviors can progress to include moderate forms of delinquency (robbery and assault) and causing harm to others. At this point, a child is said to have Conduct Disorder.

The etiology of Conduct Disorder, like that of ODD, is multifactorial. Biological studies have shown abnormalities in neurotransmitter systems, particularly noradrenergic and dopaminergic activity. Genetic studies suggest a possible heritable factor. Beyond the characteristics and temperament of the child, family factors have also been found to be important. Poor family functioning, marital problems, abusive parenting, and large family size are risk factors. Additionally, parental drug and alcohol abuse, psychiatric disorders (ADHD, and mood, psychotic, and learning disorders), and deviant or criminal activities are common factors. Given genetic loading, an abusive or neglectful home environment, and the presence of substance abuse and psychiatric co-morbidity, it's easier to understand how a child would develop a system of coping that relies on violence and intimidation.

As with ODD, the diagnosis of Conduct Disorder requires a careful assessment of the child, the family, and the child's behavior in different settings. A variety of rating scales are available, including the Conners scale and the Child Behavior Checklist. Neuropsychological testing and school records may also be helpful. Usually, we rely mainly on the clinical assessment of the child and the family and on collateral information from teachers and other significant people to get a broad view of the type and severity of behaviors, associated factors, and possible patterns of behavior. Again, the highest co-morbidity is with the other disruptive behavior disorders; 90 percent of children diagnosed with Conduct Disorder met criteria for ODD at an earlier age. The co-occurrence of Conduct Disorder and ADHD is highest in the preteen years and then decreases slightly in the teen years. Other co-morbid conditions include anxiety and mood disorders, learning disorders, and developmental disorders. Almost any condition with socially unacceptable behaviors can tempt the clinician to make a diagnosis of Conduct Disorder. However, what makes a diagnosis of Conduct Disorder more likely is purposeful, unacceptable behavior that violates the rights of others and often produces significant harm.

Treatment

Appropriate treatment of Conduct Disorder remains controversial and unproven. Several approaches have been tried, including hospitalization, medication, individual psychotherapy, group psychotherapy, and family psychotherapy.

(For more information about treatment of Conduct Disorder, please see *Treating Adolescents.*)

With appropriate treatment, much can be done to change the course of disruptive behaviors. This is one of the true rewards of working with children with such disorders. To succeed requires your close collaboration with the child, the family, the school, and any other systems with which the child is involved (including the criminal justice system if there is a history of delinquency, and social workers if there is a history of abuse or other legal issues). If our intervention is successful, we may have prevented the continued development of antisocial behavior and possible criminal activities, and fostered the development of a child who can do well in school and establish meaningful relationships with family and friends. By handling the behaviors early in life, we may also prevent future psychiatric disorders.

To see a child turn around and get back on track can be quite dramatic and inspiring. We cannot overemphasize the importance of patience, flexibility, and perseverance in achieving this end. Lulls and intermittent breaks in psychotherapy are common; you will no doubt experience feelings of anger, frustration, and disappointment. But in the end, if you hang in there, you have the opportunity to make a significant difference in a child's life.

NOTES

P. 93, *please see* Treating Adolescents: Lock, J. (1996). Disruptive behavioral disorders. In Steiner, H. (Ed.), *Treating adolescents*. San Francisco: Jossey-Bass.

P. 95, *ADHD is thought to describe 2 to 6 percent of children:* Schachar, R. (1991). Childhood hyperactivity. *Journal of Child Psychology & Psychiatry, 32*(1), 163–164.

P. 95, *It seems to affect boys more than girls at a rate of four to one:* Schachar, R. (1991), *ibid.*

P. 96, *Children of parents with ADHD seem to be twice as likely to develop ADHD:* Schachar, R. (1991), ibid.

P. 98, *Conners Behavioral Checklist:* Conners, C. K. (1969). A teacher rating scale for use in drug studies with children. *American Journal of Psychiatry, 126,* 884–888.

P. 100, *The most common medications used to treat ADHD are . . . (Ritalin) and . . . (Dexedrine):* Rapaport, J., Buchsbaum, M., Wengarten, H., Zahn, T., Ludlow, C., Bartko, J., & Mickkelson, E. J. (1980). Dextroamphetamine: Cognitive and behavioral effects in normal and hyperactive boys and normal adult males. *Archives of General Psychiatry, 37,* 933–943.

P. 105, *A relatively small minority of children grow up to have significant psychopathology:* Werry, J. S. (1992). Attention deficit hyperactivity disorder: History, terminology, and manifestations at different ages. *Psychiatric Clinics of North America, 1*(2), 297–310.

P. 107, *The continued problem . . . described in the* DSM-IV: American Psychiatric Association. (1994). *Diagnostic and statistical manual of mental disorders* (4th ed.). Washington, DC: Author, p. 91.

P. 108, *the prevalence is estimated to be 1.5 to 10 percent of the general population:* Cohen, P., Kasen, S., Brook, J., Struening, E. (1991). Diagnostic predictors of treatment patterns in a cohort of adolescents. *Journal of the American Academy of Child and Adolescent Psychiatry, 30*(6), 989–993.

P. 109, *Studies have shown that 33 percent of children may have two concurrent behavior disorders:* Keller, M., Lavori, P., Beardslee, W., Wunder, J., Schwartz, C., Roth, J., & Biederman, J. (1992). The disruptive behavioral disorder in children and adolescents: Comorbidity and clinical course. *Journal of the American Academy of Child and Adolescent Psychiatry, 31*(2), 204–209.

P. 115, *Positively reinforcing prosocial behavior . . . require a level of dedication . . . that many of these parents lack:* Tolan, P., & Guerra, N. (1994). Prevention of delinquency: Current status and issues. *Applied and Preventive Psychology, 3*, 251–273.

P. 115, *(4) establishing ways to resolve conflicts and disagreements:* Patterson, G. (1982). *Coercive family process.* Eugene, OR: Castalia.

P. 116, *although symptoms that started in childhood may continue into adolescence and adulthood in up to 14 percent of cases:* Keller, M., Lavori, P., Beardslee, W., Wunder, J., Schwartz, C., Roth, J., & Biederman, J. (1992). *ibid.*

P. 117, *It is a common reason for referral, accounting for 30 to 50 percent of referrals in some clinics:* Cohen, P., Kasen, S., Brook, J., Struening, E. (1991). *ibid.*

P. 117, *and the general prevalence is estimated to be 2 to 10 percent:* Cohen, P., Cohen, J., Kasen, S., Velez, C., Hartmark, C., Johnson, J., Rojas, M., Brook, J., & Struening, E. (1993). An epidemiological study of disorders in late childhood and adolescence: I. Age and gender-specific prevalence. *Journal of Child Psychology and Psychiatry, 34*(6) 851–867.

P. 117, *the number of girls with CD may actually be higher than reported:* Zoccolillo, M., Tremblay, R., & Vitano, F. (1996). *DSM-III-R* and *DSM-III* criteria for conduct disorder in preadolescent girls: Specific but insensitive. *Journal of the American Academy of Child and Adolescent Psychiatry, 35*(4), 461–470.

P. 118, *Eventually these behaviors can progress . . . and causing harm to others:* Loeber, R., Green, S., Lahey, B., & Christ, M. (1992). Developmental sequences in the age of onset of disruptive child behaviors. *Journal of Child and Family Studies, 1*(1), 21–41.

P. 118, *Biological studies have shown abnormalities in neurotransmitter systems:* Pliseka, S. (1988). Plasma neurochemistry in juvenile offenders. *Journal of the American Academy of Child and Adolescent Psychiatry, 27*(5), 588–594.

P. 118, *Genetic studies suggest a possible heritable factor:* Christians, K., & Medicine, S. (1977). *Biosocial bases of criminal behavior.* New York: Gardner Press.

P. 118, *family factors have also been found to be important:* Rutter, M. (1994). Family discord and conduct disorder: Cause, consequence or correlate? *Journal of Family Psychology, 8*(2), 170–186.

P. 118, *Conners scale:* Conners, C. K. (1969). *ibid.*

P. 118, *Child Behavior Checklist:* Achenbach, T., & Edelbrock, C. (1983). *Manual for Child Behavior Checklist and Revised Child Behavior Profile.* Burlington: Department of Psychiatry, University of Vermont.

P. 119, *90 percent of children diagnosed with Conduct Disorder met criteria for ODD:* Loeber, R., & Keenan, K. (1994). Interaction between conduct disorder and its premorbid conditions: Effects of age and gender. *Clinical Psychology Review, 14*(6), 497–523.

5

CONVERSION AND SOMATOFORM DISORDERS

Pamela J. Beasley and David Ray DeMaso

JULIE

Julie, eleven, was admitted to the hospital's neurology service for evaluation. Her symptom—difficulty maintaining her balance while walking—had begun gradually over the course of approximately one week and had persisted for the past several days. She had no history of medical problems except for a recent cold two weeks before, which had left her very dizzy and unable to walk steadily for several days. When Julie was admitted to the hospital, she was not able to walk without falling over. Extensive testing revealed no significant medical or neurological disorder that could account for her symptoms. Ultimately, a psychiatric consultation was requested.

Our evaluation revealed a child who was experiencing an early onset of puberty and who was under pressure from her peers to begin dating boys. In addition, her family had been under significant financial pressure lately, which had led to increased tension in the parent's marital relationship. We recommended to the neurology service that further medical testing be postponed, and we initiated a course of intensive individual therapy combined with parent guidance. As Julie explored her fears related to her new social pressures and her concerns about her parent's marriage, her symptoms quickly diminished, and she was soon able to return to school.

Students of psychology, medicine, and even philosophy have long been interested in the interactions between mind and body. As child psychiatrists at the consultation-liaison service at Children's Hospital in Boston, we frequently evaluate and treat children with complex medical and psychological disorders. The psychiatric consultant's role is to provide the patient and her family with support as well as to assist them in developing and strengthening coping strategies.

At other times, we are called in to evaluate children whose physical symptoms are unsupported by medical findings and the physical examination or whose symptoms are grossly in excess of what would be expected given the medical findings. These symptoms are sometimes part of a "psychosomatic disorder," or, in *DSM-IV* terminology, a Somatoform Disorder.

The Somatoform Disorders are a group of psychological disorders in which the patient experiences physical symptoms despite the absence of a neurological or "general medical" condition that would explain their presence. In no other psychological disorders are the complex interactions between mind and body more apparent than in the Somatoform Disorders. In this chapter, we will discuss important aspects of the evaluation and treatment of Somatoform Disorders in the preschool and school-age population. Please refer to *Treating Adolescents* for a description of these disorders in the adolescent population.

Somatoform Disorders are most frequently diagnosed by mental health clinicians who work within a medical setting such as a hospital or outpatient pediatric clinic. Thus, it is especially important for mental health clinicians in these settings to be able to recognize these disorders, so as to prevent invasive, expensive, and often unnecessary medical workups.

There are a total of five major diagnoses that fall under the heading of the Somatoform Disorders. These include Conversion Disorder, Somatization Disorder, Pain Disorder, Hypochondriasis, and Body Dysmorphic Disorder. Because Hypochondriasis and Body Dysmorphic Disorder are extremely rare in the preschool and school-age populations, we do not discuss them in this chapter.

CONVERSION DISORDER

FRANK

Frank was a previously physically healthy eight-year-old boy who developed the inability to walk over a period of four weeks. Repeated physical examinations were normal, as were X-rays of his leg and hip. Consultation with specialists from orthopedics and neurology found normal examinations. The presenting symptoms were not explained by an apparent medical disorder. Frank's pediatrician next requested a psychiatric consultation.

A psychiatric interview with Frank and his parents revealed a pre-morbidly emotionally healthy boy with a tendency to have heightened somatic complaints. Significant losses in this same time period included his parents' separating and the death of a close paternal grandfather. His grandfather had been immobilized over the past six months related to progressive amyotrophic lateral sclerosis.

The prior history of somatic complaints, the temporally related family stresses, and the symptom model, combined with symptoms unexplained by a general medical condition, supported the diagnosis of a Conversion Disorder.

In DSM-IV, Conversion Disorder is characterized by one or more symptoms affecting voluntary motor or sensory function that suggest a neurological or other general medical condition. Psychological factors are judged to be associated with the symptom because the initiation or exacerbation of the symptom is preceded by conflicts or stressors. The symptom is not intentionally produced or feigned. After appropriate investigation, the symptom cannot be fully explained by a medical condition, by the direct effects of a substance, or as a culturally sanctioned behavior. Conversion Disorder causes clinically significant distress or impairment in social or academic functioning.

In children, conversion symptoms typically occur suddenly and temporarily. Typical sensory losses include blindness, deafness, loss of touch, pain sensation, and diplopia. Motor symptoms include paralysis, ataxia, aphonia, dysphagia, urinary retention, and seizures. Pseudoseizures ("emotional" or "nonepileptic" seizures), unexplained falls, and episodes of fainting are the most common abnormalities, followed by gait and sensory deficits.

In these cases it is important to determine whether there is a history of psychological stress or trauma. Through your interview, you can look for a temporal relationship between the stressor(s) and the development of the conversion symptom. Additionally you want to note whether there is a prior history of conversion symptoms or recurrent somatic complaints. Recent family stress, unresolved grief reactions, and family psychopathology occur at a higher frequency in children with conversion symptoms. The presence of a symptom model (for example, a family member with similar deficits) is also helpful in making the diagnosis. Patients with pseudoseizures have been found to have significant prior histories of trauma, especially sexual abuse. La belle indifference and histrionic personality traits, once thought in the adult literature to be characteristic of these patients, have not proven to be reliable diagnostic criteria in children. The following list summarizes the important interview criteria for diagnosis of Conversion Disorder:

- Psychological stress temporally related to symptom
- Prior history of conversion symptoms
- Prior history of recurrent somatic complaints
- Dissociative or somatization disorders, or both
- Family stress or psychopathology, or both
- Symptom model

SUSAN

Susan, six, was admitted to the neurology service for evaluation of episodes in which her arms and legs would shake violently for five to ten minutes at a time. Susan was admitted in order to rule out a seizure disorder, and her symptoms were carefully monitored while she was in the hospital. The neurologists were unable to find brain wave abnormalities corresponding to her seizure-like episodes, and we were brought in to consult.

In the course of our evaluation, we learned that the onset of her symptoms had been proceeded by a previously undisclosed episode of sexual abuse by a male baby-sitter. We were able to determine that Susan's symptoms served to keep her mother close in order to provide safety. After we reported the episode of abuse to the family and the Department of Social Services and initiated counseling, the symptoms rapidly subsided.

On physical examination, Conversion Disorder symptoms do not conform to known anatomical pathways and physiological mechanisms, and if physical findings are present they may relate either to muscle atrophy from disuse or to sequelae of medical procedures. There are no specific laboratory studies associated with Conversion Disorder. Video-electroencephalographic monitoring has been increasingly used to investigate seizure disorders. The lack of brain wave abnormalities in association with seizure-like behavior makes pseudoseizures or Conversion Disorder a likely diagnosis. Psychological tests including neuropsychological testing and projective testing can be helpful in adding to the evidence for Conversion Disorder, though they cannot confirm the diagnosis.

Epidemiology

In most studies, the incidence of Conversion Disorder varies between 0.5 and 10 percent. It is three times more common in adolescents than preadolescents and very rarely occurs in children under five years of age. It is more common in girls during adolescence and is equally distributed among school-age boys and girls.

Conversion symptoms typically occur suddenly and are of short duration. Pediatricians are most likely to see children with transient reactions, whereas psychiatrists tend to be consulted in the more difficult cases where symptoms have become more protracted. Symptoms may become chronic or recurrent, especially when the precipitating stress is persistent or repetitive, when there is associated significant psychopathology, or when the symptom provides significant secondary gain. Patients with pseudoseizures are more likely to have recurrences than patients with paralysis or aphonia, and although early studies suggested that significant percentages of children with an initial diagnosis of Conversion Disorder were subsequently found to have a medical illness, more recent samples have revealed a more modest risk (less than 10 percent) of faulty diagnosis in children.

Etiology

According to psychodynamic theory, Conversion Disorder symptoms are direct symbolic expressions of an underlying psychological conflict. The unconscious conflict is "converted" to a somatic symptom. The patient is said to achieve "primary gain" by keeping the conflict from consciousness and as a result minimizing anxiety. The symptom can provide "secondary gain" to the patient by allowing an escape from unwanted consequences or responsibilities.

It is not unusual for a child to quickly learn the benefits of assuming the sick role. Increased parental attention and avoidance of unpleasant school pressures may only further reinforce her symptom. Physical symptoms have been viewed as a form of body language in children who have difficulty expressing their emotions verbally. For example, we frequently see children with Conversion Disorder who have difficulties disclosing abuse or expressing their anger. Likewise, high-achieving children who cannot admit they are under too much pressure may present with conversion symptoms. And social learning theory suggests that some symptoms are a result of modeling or observational learning within a family.

In fact, family systems play important roles in initiating and maintaining symptoms. Minuchin described four specific family transactional patterns that can be associated with Conversion Disorder: enmeshment, overprotectiveness, rigidity, and lack of conflict resolution. A central focus on the illness often allows the avoidance of conflict within the family, which can reinforce the child's illness behavior.

Differential Diagnosis

As the child's clinician, your major diagnostic concern is the exclusion of neurological or general medical conditions. Migraine syndromes, temporal lobe epilepsy, and central nervous system tumors have presented difficult diagnostic dilemmas. You also need to be alert to the dual existence of a medical condition and Conversion Disorder (for example, seizures and pseudoseizures in the same patient).

According to the *DSM-IV,* the essential feature of Psychological Factors Affecting Medical Condition is the presence of one or more specific psychological or behavioral factors that adversely affect a general medical condition. Personality traits, coping style, maladaptive health behaviors, a mental disorder, or stress-related physiological responses are different psychological factors that can have an impact on a general medical condition. This is in contrast to Conversion Disorder, in which no medical condition exists to completely account for the symptoms produced.

Depressive, anxiety, and stress disorders can all present with symptoms similar to Conversion Disorder. However, Conversion Disorder should not be diagnosed if the symptoms are better accounted for by these disorders. You need to identify the presence of disabling depression or anxiety that has been present for over two weeks and that began prior to the development of the conversion symptom.

Conversion symptoms can also occur in the course of Somatization Disorder, Pain Disorder, and Factitious Disorder by Proxy. In Somatization Disorder, there is a multiple-symptom pattern in contrast to monosymptomatic and usually time-limited Conversion Disorder presentation. Pain Disorder is diagnosed if the symptoms are limited to pain. Factitious Disorder Not Otherwise Specified, or Munchausen syndrome by proxy, is a perpetrator's production of symptoms in another person who is under the individual's care. This syndrome is most often present in the preschool-age population. The motivation for the perpetrator's behavior is presumed to be a psychological need to assume a sick role. You need to maintain an index of suspicion and take a thorough history to make the diagnosis.

You must also keep in mind that physical changes resembling conversion symptoms are common aspects of certain culturally sanctioned religious and healing rituals. Falling down with loss or alteration of consciousness is a feature of a variety of culture-specific syndromes.

Treatment

You need to evaluate the biological, psychiatric, and social dimensions both separately and in relation to each other in all Somatoform Disorders. Given the common "diagnostic uncertainty" in these disorders with frequent dual medical-psychiatric diagnoses, we strongly recommend an integrated medical and psychiatric treatment program. A combined approach sidesteps the "organic versus psychiatric" dilemma that clinicians often face. Table 5.1 provides an outline of this integrated approach to evaluation and treatment.

The Pediatrician's Role. The child and family generally present to their pediatrician with concern about a medical cause for the problem. The pediatrician begins the assessment with an exploration of both medical and psychological factors that may be contributing to the clinical presentation. In many cases that are associated with significant emotional factors, reassurance and suggestion from the pediatrician that the symptom will improve

Table 5.1
The Components of an Integrated Medical and Psychiatric Approach for Children and Adolescents with Somatoform Disorders

Psychiatry evaluation
   Elicit diagnostic criteria
   Facilitate consolidation or better understanding of experience by family
Formulation
   Understand patient from biopsychosocial perspective
   Integrate psychiatric formulation with pediatrician
Informing conference
   Family has medical model as frame of reference
   Join with pediatrician to reframe understanding of symptoms
Interventions
   Medical
      Ongoing pediatric follow-up
      Physical therapy as needed
   Psychiatric
      Psychotherapy
      Cognitive-behavioral therapy
      Family therapy
      Psychopharmacology

---

are helpful. However, in more complicated cases psychiatric referral is indicated.

The pediatrician can facilitate the evaluation by establishing close communication with you. The family can be told by the pediatrician that she is requesting a consultation as part of a full evaluation that includes all aspects of the child. The pediatrician should not send the family away but rather communicate that she will integrate your findings into a comprehensive understanding of the child's symptoms.

Evaluation and Formulation. As the mental health clinician, you should take a full history and mental status examination, being alert to the areas we highlighted in the previous clinical interview section. In addition, it is important to pay close attention to the patient's "story." Telling you this story will frequently allow the family to consolidate or better understand their experience. You can begin to understand the clinical presentation "in the family's own words."

Your formulation of the problem is crucial. Families often believe that the symptom picture is due solely to a medical condition. This view of the problem needs to be reframed with a biopsychosocial understanding, which should then be communicated to the pediatrician. You need to be alert to the frustration engendered in physicians by these patients, as physicians may not see them as "deserving" of the sick role. Other reactions have included dismissing the patient as being "hysterical" or pursuing the "million-dollar workup."

Conference. The next step is an "informing conference" that includes the pediatrician and family. In this meeting, you present the significant psychological aspects of the case to the patient and family in a supportive and nonjudgmental manner. The family should be told that many important things have been discovered; for example, "We have good news: we have ruled out a number of serious illnesses." You should avoid such statements as "We couldn't find anything," "It's in your mind," or "The symptoms are not real." Close attention to the family's words and way of thinking allows for their words to be integrated into a more biopsychosocial formulation, thereby facilitating family acceptance.

Treatment Team. Following the family's acceptance of a new formulation of the problem, you can facilitate the formation of a medical-psychiatric team. This team supports both your interventions and the pediatrician's ongoing monitoring and treatment for possible medical illness. The pediatrician can provide ongoing follow-up while avoiding unnecessary medical investigations and procedures. Many patients benefit from physical therapy that enables a graduated return to the child's usual activities.

Treatment Plan. We then create for each family a clearly identified solution-focused treatment plan directed toward understanding the child and family's dynamics and the child's reasons for assuming the sick role. We integrate a number of theoretical perspectives including cognitive, behavioral, psychoeducational, psychodynamic, family, group, developmental, and biological approaches into a practical intervention program. The goal is to help the child and family develop a coping approach. This approach allows us to provide the effective, efficient, and well-defined intervention programs that are crucial when requesting insurance coverage from a family's carrier.

Potential interventions include individual, behavioral, cognitive, family, and pharmacological therapies. Children with high levels of psychological insight can benefit from individual psychotherapy. Psychodynamically oriented therapy may be helpful in identifying unconscious conflicts that may be maintaining symptoms. You can facilitate the expression of feelings and encourage more adaptive coping mechanisms.

Behavioral modification techniques are common interventions, especially in families who are less psychologically minded. The therapy should be aimed at reinforcing health-related behaviors and diminishing illness responses. You can use such techniques as hypnosis, biofeedback, and relaxation training to teach the patient control over certain physiological processes, such as autonomic system activity. Cognitive therapy can be helpful in identifying negative, maladaptive thoughts or emotions that can contribute to an increase in the degree of pain, suffering, and disability.

Family Therapy. Family therapy and parent guidance are important components of any treatment program. Family therapy should explore ways in which the child's symptoms may serve to stabilize the family system (for example, how focus on the symptoms allows for avoidance of conflict). The family should be discouraged from reinforcing the symptoms, and they should learn ways of providing positive reinforcement for improvement of functioning. The child should be assisted in abandoning the sick role through the encouragement of developmentally appropriate activities that can lead to a sense of mastery.

It is not uncommon for families to remain resistant to psychiatric intervention. In these cases it is helpful for you to remain a consultant to the pediatrician, providing advice about ways in which the physician can decrease reinforcement of the sick role and encourage mobilization of the patient. You can also advise regarding the need for social service intervention around possible parental neglect or abuse (such as seeking multiple unnecessary medical procedures).

OTHER SOMATOFORM DISORDERS

We are often called about another group of youngsters with multiple physical symptoms that cannot be readily explained by their pediatricians. These symptoms are particularly frustrating to the physicians and very upsetting to the parents.

JILL

Nine-year-old Jill had not felt well for over nine months. When she came to us for evaluation, she complained of generalized weakness and fatigue. She had shown evidence of strep throat in the beginning of her illness, but subsequent evaluations were normal. Additional medical workups by nearly a half dozen specialists found no general medical condition that could account for her symptoms.

Prior to the onset of her symptoms, Jill was described as a remarkable girl with excellent grades as well as outstanding performances as a gymnast and violinist. Her parents noted that she had good friendships, though she was often viewed as intensely competitive. A conflicted relationship between her professional parents had improved at the same time that her symptoms had continued. Jill's mother had a long history of multiple somatic complaints involving multiple organ systems.

Jill's long-standing unexplained somatic complaints and positive family history for recurrent somatic complaints, combined with the possible secondary gains of avoiding high expectations and reducing parental conflict supported our diagnosis of Undifferentiated Somatoform Disorder.

Presentation

According to the *DSM-IV*, an essential feature of Somatization Disorder is a pattern of recurring, multiple, and clinically significant complaints. Pain, gastrointestinal, sexual-reproductive, and pseudoneurological symptoms are all required for the diagnosis, and these complaints cannot be explained by any known medical condition. The complaint is considered to be clinically significant if it results in medical treatment, causes impairment in functioning, or both.

Obviously, the number of symptoms required over a several-year period and the inclusion of a required sexual symptom mitigate against the diagnosis being made in prepubertal children. Therefore, children are more likely to meet *DSM-IV* criteria for Undifferentiated Somatoform Disorder; these criteria require only one or more unexplained physical complaint(s), functional impairment, and a duration of six months. Symptoms of less than six months are coded in *DSM-IV* as Somatoform Disorder Not Otherwise Specified.

The most frequent complaints of clients with Somatization Disorder are chronic fatigue, loss of appetite, or gastrointestinal-genitourinary symptoms. "Neurasthenia," which is characterized by fatigue and weakness, is classified in the *DSM-IV* as Undifferentiated Somatoform Disorder. This latter syndrome is historically quite similar to "chronic fatigue syndrome," which has been a focus of attention over the past decade. There is often a history of treatment from many physicians concurrently. Comorbid symptoms of anxiety and depression are common.

As with Conversion Disorder, the symptoms do not conform to known physiological mechanisms. If physical signs are present they relate most often to the sequelae of medical procedures.

The absence of laboratory findings is characteristic. Psychological testing may be useful in understanding the individual, though it cannot confirm a diagnosis. The Children's Somatization Inventory has been used in some studies to identify children at risk. The measure is a list of thirty-six somatic symptoms derived from the *DSM-III's* Somatization Disorder criteria.

Epidemiology

Although childhood somatic complaints are not uncommon, the diagnosis of Somatization Disorder is rarely made before adulthood, with the majority of cases beginning in adolescence. The *DSM-IV* criteria for Undifferentiated Somatoform Disorder are new, so the epidemiology is uncertain. However, child and adolescent "somatic complaints syndromes" have been reported in studies with prevalence rates ranging from 4.5 to 15 percent.

The outcome for patients with recurrent somatic complaints is less positive when follow-up assessment includes global emotional functioning as opposed to only measuring whether the original symptom is present or absent. Pseudoneurological symptoms may be especially predictive of later functional disability. Chronic fatigue syndrome appears to be a nonprogressive disease with a general trend for improvement, if not complete recovery.

Etiology

The severity and frequency of the somatic symptoms can be understood through application of the psychodynamic, learning, and family system theories discussed earlier in relation to Conversion Disorder.

Adoption studies have shown that genetic factors may contribute to the development of the Somatization Disorder. Studies have also found evidence for a relationship between this disorder and Attention Deficit Hyperactivity Disorder (ADHD). Somatization Disorder is observed in 10 to 20 percent of female first-degree relatives of patients with ADHD. Having a male or female relative with antisocial personality increases the risk for development of Somatization Disorder.

A "hysterical" information-processing pattern characterized by distractibility, difficulty distinguishing target and nontarget stimuli, and impaired verbal communication has been found in individuals with Somatization Disorder. This pattern or deficit has been postulated to underlie the frequent physical complaints along with the vague and circumstantial processing of social and personal problems. This pattern has not been shown in children. Children who present with multiple somatic symptoms often seem to have a striking absence of vocabulary to describe emotions. Somatic symptoms have been referred to as "body language" for emotional expression.

Differential Diagnosis

One of the challenges you face early on when assessing children for Somatoform Disorders is the fact that these disorders share many of the same symptoms as other disorders. For example, you will need to rule out medical illnesses with vague and multiple somatic symptoms (for example, acute intermittent porphyria, hypercalcemia, or collagen vascular diseases). Also, chronic fatigue syndrome is characterized by the onset of persistent or relapsing debilitating fatigue, which often follows an acute infection. The fatigue impairs daily activity for at least six months and cannot be explained by either medical or psychiatric illness. Additional symptoms may include muscle weakness, headaches, mild fever, painful adenopathy, and migratory arthralgia. Depression and anxiety-related symptoms are common in this syndrome. Viral infections, immune dysfunction, and neuropsychologic problems are either inciting or perpetuating factors. The syndrome is most likely a result of multiple etiologies of which one is an Undifferentiated Somatoform Disorder.

As noted previously, depressive disorders can be accompanied by multiple somatic complaints. Recurrent Panic Attacks and Generalized Anxiety Disorder may be difficult to distinguish from somatoform disorders. Symptoms associated with depressive and anxiety disorders encompass a broader range of complaints. In contrast, Somatoform Disorders have a focused and primary concern with somatic complaints. Nevertheless, these other disorders may be co-morbid with Somatoform Disorders.

Treatment

There is no single optimal treatment of an Undifferentiated Somatoform Disorder. The integrated medical and psychiatric approach previously described is also applicable for these disorders (see Table 5.1). The number of doctors, as well as the number of diagnostic evaluations and treatments, should be limited. Your treatment and attention should be directed toward personal and social problems rather than somatic complaints. Prescription medications need to be kept at a minimum. If there are co-morbid anxiety or depressive disorders, appropriate psychotropic medications can be considered. Everyone involved needs to maintain firm limits on excessive or manipulative demands from the patient.

Finally, it is important to remember that cases identified in childhood may represent the earliest presentation of a lifelong pattern of disabling somatoform symptoms. Although there is no supporting research to confirm this, aggressive intervention is indicated before the child establishes an ingrained "sick role." Multimodal interventions including psychotherapy, cognitive-behavioral methods, family therapy, and inpatient psychiatry admission have all been used in the treatment, depending on the formulation of the problems in each individual case.

PAIN DISORDER

We see a number of children and adolescents for whom pain is the predominant focus of their presentation. These youngsters can present with much distress and disability and yet have no clear medical condition to account for the severity of their pain. They are often referred to us with an urgency for intervention and pain relief.

JOSHUA

Joshua was a nine-year-old boy admitted to the medical service to evaluate his recurrent abdominal pain and nausea. A thorough workup had failed to reveal a medical etiology for his chronic pain and nausea, so a psychiatric referral was made. On examination, Joshua presented as a highly anxious boy who was under a great deal of pressure from his professional parents to excel academically. Psychoeducational testing revealed a previously undetected learning disability that was impinging on his ability to perform academically. A comprehensive treatment program including cognitive-behavioral techniques to reduce his anxiety, tutoring to enhance his learning skills, guidance for his parents, and ongoing medical follow-up resulted in a rapid reduction in Joshua's symptoms of abdominal pain and nausea.

In *DSM-IV,* pain of sufficient severity to warrant clinical attention is the primary criteria for Pain Disorder. The pain must be of sufficient severity to cause significant distress or impairment in social, school, or home functioning. Psychological factors are deemed to play an important role in the onset, severity, exacerbation, or maintenance of the pain. The pain is not intentionally produced or feigned, nor can the pain be better accounted for by another psychiatric disorder.

Pain disorders are divided into two subtypes: (1) Pain Disorder Associated With Psychological Factors, in which emotional factors alone are judged to play a major role; and (2) Pain Disorder Associated With Both Psychological Factors and a General Medical Condition, in which both together are deemed to have important roles in the onset, severity, exacerbation, or maintenance of the pain. Each subtype of Pain Disorder is further classified as either acute (duration of less than six months) or chronic (duration of more than six months). Pain that is judged to be entirely related to a general medical condition is not considered a psychiatric disorder and is coded on *DSM-IV's* Axis III.

Epidemiology

Recurrent complaints of pain appear quite commonly in children and adolescents. Headaches, recurrent abdominal pain, limb pain, and chest pain have been reported with prevalence rates ranging from 7 to 30 percent in both community and clinical samples. The prevalence of Pain Disorder in children and adolescents as defined by *DSM-IV* remains to be documented in the literature.

Etiology

Psychodynamic theory holds that the defense mechanism of conversion underlies medically unexplained pain. *Conversion* refers to the transformation of repressed affect related to psychic conflict from the emotional realm to the physical one. Unconscious conflicts are symbolically represented by the pain. The symptom of pain can serve the unconscious goal of removing the individual from a conflictual situation as well as representing an unconscious form of self-punishment for unacceptable feelings.

The concept of a "pain-prone patient or disorder" postulates that there are individuals with histories of childhood abuse or neglect who develop pain that is related to underlying feelings of guilt, depression, aggression, or loss. Engel proposed that the experience of childhood abuse led to internalization of pain, association of pain with badness, and subsequent use of pain to alleviate feelings of guilt related to aggressive impulses toward the parent.

There are no unifying biological explanations for pain disorders. The neurobiological components of pain involve complex interactions between ascending and descending pain pathways within the central and peripheral nervous systems. Endorphins and biogenic amine neurotransmitters such as serotonin and norepinephrine play important modulating roles in descending pain pathways. Drugs (such as antidepressants) that potentiate the central effects of biogenic amines have been useful in producing analgesia by increasing their concentrations in these descending pathways. Studies have shown that the concentrations of serotonin and endorphin metabolites are reduced in the spinal fluid of patients with chronic pain.

Chronic pain often causes decreased mobility and poor posture, which may result in the development of pathological changes such as osteoporosis, contractures, myofibrositis, and circulatory and respiratory disturbances. These conditions often lead to stimulation of peripheral afferent fibers, creating a "vicious cycle of progressive deterioration."

Classical and operant conditioning can lead to the perpetuation of pain-related behaviors long after the initial noxious stimulus has been removed. Classical conditioning results from the repeated pairing of a neutral, or conditioned, stimulus with an unconditioned stimulus that evokes a response, such that the neutral stimulus eventually comes to evoke the response. For example, settings that have been associated with pain may alone trigger pain-related behavior.

Operant conditioning holds that behaviors which are rewarded will increase in strength or frequency, whereas behaviors that are inhibited or punished will decrease. Pain-related behaviors may be reinforced by attention and sympathy from others, the euphoric effects of pain medications, and a decrease in responsibilities. If the pain behaviors or responses are reinforced early on in the course of the pain disorder, then it is likely that these behaviors will continue even after removal of the original painful stimulus. Conversely, health-related behaviors will diminish, as they are no longer subject to systematic reinforcement.

Many studies have investigated the role of the family in the development of pain disorders. The following factors within a family have been found to be associated with these disorders: somatic preoccupation, recurrent pain complaints, alcohol abuse, and psychological disorder. Social learning theory suggests that the pain symptoms are a result of modeling or observational learning within the family. Minuchin described four specific family transactional patterns that can relate to pain disorders: enmeshment, overprotectiveness, rigidity, and lack of conflict resolution. Focus on the child's illness allows for avoidance of conflict within the family, which can reinforce the child's illness behavior.

Studies investigating the effects of ethnicity on pain tolerance and behavior have yielded mixed results. For example, some empirical studies report that Irish and Anglo-Saxons have greater pain tolerance than individuals of southern Mediterranean ethnicity, whereas others have found no significant differences among ethnic groups.

Diagnosis

It is important to perform a thorough psychiatric interview when assessing a child for all Somatoform Disorders. You must determine whether the child has a major psychiatric disorder, and you need to evaluate whether there are etiological factors associated with the child's pain symptoms. Finally, you need to evaluate if these symptoms exist simultaneously with a pain syndrome, are secondary to a medical disorder, or exist independently and are etiologic to the pain syndrome.

You need to pay close attention to both current and past psychosocial stressors, in particular noting whether pain seems to be situation-dependent or temporally related to a stressor. You should obtain the history of prior episodes of pain in the patient as well as of pain syndromes in other family members.

In the case of Pain Disorder, the symptoms are neuroanatomically inconsistent with known pathways or are grossly in excess of what would be expected from the physical findings. If physical findings are present, they are secondary to pathological changes associated with immobilization.

There are no specific laboratory abnormalities associated with pain disorders. Infrared thermography may be helpful in identifying changes in temperature and vascular flow associated with certain disorders that can cause chronic pain.

The Minnesota Multiphasic Personality Inventory (MMPI) has been used in the diagnostic evaluation of adults with chronic pain, and it typically reveals elevations in the hypochondriasis and hysteria scales. The Personality Inventory for Children has been used for similar diagnostic purposes; however, its ability to differentiate between organic symptoms and conversion symptoms is in question.

Differential Diagnosis

Every child and adolescent has a psychological reaction to experienced pain. The diagnosis of disorder is made when the response is out of proportion to the general medical condition and when deficits or impairment in emotional and behavioral functioning occur.

Important medical causes of pain that can be confused with psychogenic pain disorders include reflex sympathetic dystrophy, headache syndromes, myofascial pain, posttraumatic syndromes, neuropathy, and tumors.

Pain and depression frequently occur together. Some researchers have suggested that Pain Disorder may be a variant of depression. Lesse coined the term *masked depression* to refer to clinical presentations in which pain is the primary complaint. The potential demoralization and learned helplessness experienced with pain may lead to depressive symptoms. Pain disorders should only be diagnosed if the symptoms cannot be better accounted for by depressive disorders or if the symptoms are in excess of those associated with depression.

Pain symptoms commonly occur in the course of Somatization Disorder. The latter is diagnosed usually in adulthood and is accompanied by a history of symptom development often beginning in adolescence. Conversion Disorder refers to medically unexplained deficits in motor and sensory functioning; it is often accompanied by pain symptoms. Patients commonly experience conversion and pain symptoms together.

Malingering involves the intentional production or feigning of symptoms. The motivation for the behavior is the conscious goal of gaining or avoiding something in the environment, for example, avoiding criminal prosecution or seeking financial gain. Generally, this diagnosis is rarely seen in children, though occasionally an older adolescent with antisocial traits may present with somatic symptoms.

Factitious Disorder is characterized by physical symptoms that are intentionally produced or feigned in order to assume the sick role. This disorder is generally described in adults, though some older children and adolescent cases have been reported. As discussed earlier, Factitious Disorder by Proxy, or Munchausen syndrome by proxy, is a perpetrator's production of symptoms in another person who is under the individual's care. This syndrome most often presents with preschool children as the patient. The motivation for the perpetrator's behavior is presumed to be a psychological need to assume a sick role. You need to maintain an index of suspicion and take a thorough history to make the diagnosis.

Course

There has been little written about the course of Pain Disorder in children. Follow-up studies with patients with recurrent abdominal pain found that 25 to 50 percent continue to suffer abdominal discomfort in adulthood. Course of illness has been related to associated psychopathology, duration of pain, and extent of environmental reinforcement.

Treatment

As described previously, the integrated medical and psychiatric approach is useful in the treatment of Pain Disorder, as it is for all Somatoform Disorders (see Table 5.1). There have been no significant controlled trials of therapy described for these disorders.

Unexplained somatic complaints in children represent a significant challenge to you and your pediatric colleagues. Physical symptoms are not simply caused by medical conditions but can also be influenced by a child's emotions, thoughts, and environment. Somatization describes a process in which a child and family seek medical help for symptoms that are misattributed to physical disease. Unexplained physical symptoms are common and problematic in many pediatric practices. Many of these complaints are transient symptoms that do not reach levels of psychiatric disorder. Nevertheless, some children have symptoms that can become quite disabling and impairing and that may represent the onset of chronic disorder. For these reasons, it is crucial that mental health clinicians be proficient in the diagnosis and treatment of this spectrum of disorders.

NOTES

P. 124, *Please refer to* Treating Adolescents: Collier, J. A. (1996). Chronic illness and somatization. In Steiner, H. (Ed.), *Treating adolescents* (pp. 261–307). San Francisco: Jossey-Bass.

P. 124, *There are a total of five major diagnoses:* American Psychiatric Association. (1994). *Diagnostic and statistical manual of mental disorders* (4th ed.). Washington, DC: Author, pp. 445–469.

P. 125, *In DSM-IV, Conversion Disorder is characterized:* American Psychiatric Association. (1994). *ibid.*, pp. 452–457.

P. 126, *followed by gait and sensory deficits:* Campo, J. V., & Fritsch, S. L. (1994). Somatization in children and adolescents. *Journal of the American Academy of Child and Adolescent Psychiatry, 33,* 1223–1235.

P. 126, *in children with conversion symptoms:* Maloney, M. J. (1980). Diagnosing hysterical conversion reactions in children. *Journal of Pediatrics, 97,* 1016–1020.

P. 126, *is also helpful in making the diagnosis:* Cloninger, C. R. (1994). Somatoform and dissociative disorders. In G. Winokur & P. J. Clayton (Eds.), *The medical basis of psychiatry* (2nd ed., pp. 169–192). Philadelphia: Saunders.

P. 126, *Patients with pseudoseizures have been found:* Bowman, E. S., & Markand, O. N. (1996). Psychodynamics and psychiatric diagnoses of pseudoseizure subjects. *American Journal of Psychiatry, 153,* 57–63.

P. 127, *The lack of brain wave abnormalities in association with seizure:* Nemzer, E. D. (1991). Somatoform Disorders. In M. Lewis (Ed.), *Child and adolescent psychiatry: A comprehensive textbook* (pp. 697–707). Baltimore: Williams & Wilkins.

P. 127, *In most studies, the incidence of Conversion Disorder:* Woodbury, M. M., DeMaso, D. R., & Goldman, S. J. (1992). An integrated medical and psychiatric approach to conversion symptoms in a four-year-old. *Journal of the American Academy of Child Adolescent Psychiatry 31,* 1095–1097.

P. 128, *or when the symptom provides significant secondary gain:* Cloninger, C. R. (1994). *ibid.*

P. 128, *patients with paralysis or aphonia:* Hafeiz, H. B. (1980). Hysterical conversion: A prognostic study. *British Journal of Psychiatry, 136,* 548–551; Weintraub, M. I. (1983). *Hysterical conversion reactions: A clinical guide to diagnosis and treatment.* New York: Spectrum.

P. 128, *although early studies suggested . . . subsequently found to have a medical illness:* Ramsay, A. R. (1984). The relationship of pathogenic mechanisms to treatment in patients with pain. *Psychotherapeutics and Psychosomatics, 42,* 69–79.

P. 128, *more recent sample have revealed . . . of faulty diagnosis in children:* Campo, J. V., & Fritsch, S. L. (1994). *ibid.*

P. 128, *have difficulty expressing emotions verbally:* Nemzer, E. D. (1991). *ibid.*

P. 128, *and social learning theory suggests . . . observational learning within a family:* Jamison, R. N., & Walker, L. S. (1992). Illness behavior in children of chronic pain patients. *International Journal of Psychiatry in Medicine, 22,* 329–342.

P. 129, *Minuchin described four specific family transactional patterns . . . Conversion Disorder:* Minuchin, S., Baker, L., Rosman, B. L., et al. (1975). A conceptual model of psychosomatic illness in children. *Archives of General Psychiatry, 32,* 1031–1038.

P. 129, *According to the DSM-IV, the essential feature of Psychological Factors Affecting Medical Condition:* American Psychiatric Association. (1994). *ibid.*

P. 130, *Factitious Disorder Not Otherwise Specified, or Munchausen syndrome by proxy, . . . under the individual's care:* American Psychiatric Association. (1994). *ibid;* Schreier, H. A., & Libow, J. A. (1993). *Hurting for love: Munchausen by proxy syndrome.* New York: Guilford Press.

P. 130, *This syndrome is most often present in the preschool-age population:* Rosenberg, D. A. (1987). Web of deceit: A literature review of Munchausen by proxy syndrome. *Child Abuse and Neglect, 11,* 547–563.

P. 130, *Falling down with loss or alteration of consciousness is a feature of a variety of culture-specific syndromes:* American Psychiatric Association. (1994). *ibid.*

P. 130, *evaluate the biological, psychiatric, and social dimensions both separately and in relation to each other in all Somatoform Disorders:* Richtesmeier, A. J., & Aschkenasy, J. R. (1988). Psychological consultation and psychosomatic diagnosis. *Psychosomatics, 29,* 338–341.

P. 130, *reassurance and suggestion from the pediatrician that the symptom will improve are helpful:* Nemzer, E. D. (1991). *ibid.*

P. 132, *Other reactions have included dismissing the patient as being "hysterical" or pursuing the "million-dollar workup.":* Stinnett, J. L. (1987). The functional somatic symptom. *Psychiatric Clinics of North America, 10,* 19–33.

P. 132, *This team supports both your interventions . . . and treatment for possible medical illness:* Ramsay, A. R. (1984). *ibid.*

P. 133, *The goal is to help the child and family develop a coping approach:* Stinnett, J. L. (1987). *ibid.*

P. 133, *Behavioral modification techniques are common interventions, . . . who are less psychologically minded:* Woodbury, M. M., DeMaso, D. R., & Goldman, S. J. (1992). *ibid.*

P. 133, *Cognitive therapy can be helpful in identifying negative, maladaptive thoughts or emotions:* Turner, J. A., & Romano, J. M. (1989). Cognitive-behavioral therapy for chronic pain patients. In J. D. Loeser & K. J. Egan (Eds.), *Managing the chronic pain patient* (pp. 95–104). New York: Raven Press.

P. 135, *According to the* DSM-IV, *an essential feature of Somatization Disorder:* American Psychiatric Association. (1994). *ibid.*, pp. 446–450.

P. 135, *Undifferentiated Somatoform Disorder:* American Psychiatric Association. (1994). *ibid.*, pp. 450–452.

P. 135, *or gastrointestinal-genitourinary symptoms:* American Psychiatric Association. (1994). *ibid.*

P. 136, *"chronic fatigue syndrome," which has been a focus of attention over the past decade:* Dale, J. K., & Straus, S. E. (1992). The chronic fatigue syndrome: Considerations relevant to children and adolescents. *Advances in Pediatric Infectious Disease, 7,* 63–83.

P. 136, *The Children's Somatization Inventory:* Walker, L. S., & Greene, J. W. (1989). Children with recurrent abdominal pain and their parents: More somatic complaints, anxiety and depression than other families? *Journal of Pediatric Psychology, 14,* 231–243; Walker, L. S., Garber, J., & Greene, J. W. (1991). Somatization symptoms in pediatric abdominal pain patients: Relation to chronicity of abdominal pain and parent somatization. *Journal of Abnormal Child Psychology, 19,* 379–394.

P. 136, *used in some studies to identify children at risk:* Garber, J., Walker, L. S., & Zeman, J. (1991). Somatization symptoms in a community sample of children and adolescents: Further validation of the Children's Somatization Inventory. *Psychological Assessment: A Journal of Consulting and Clinical Psychology, 3,* 588–595.

P. 136, DSM III*'s Somatization Disorder criteria:* American Psychiatric Association. (1980). *Diagnostic and statistical manual of mental disorders* (3rd ed.). Washington, DC: Author.

P. 136, *"somatic complaints syndromes" have been reported in studies with prevalence rates ranging from 4.5 to 15 percent:* Achenbach, T. M., Conners, C. K., Quay, H. C., Verhulst, F. C., & Howell, C. T. (1989). Replication of empirically derived syndromes as a basis for taxonomy of child/adolescent psychopathology. *Journal of Abnormal Child Psychology, 17,* 299–323; Garrick, T., Ostrov, E., & Offer, D. (1988). Physical symptoms and self-image in a group of normal adolescents. *Psychosomatics, 29,* 73–80; Offord, D. R., Boyle, M. H., Szatmari, P., et al. (1987). Ontario Child Health Study: II.

Six-month prevalence of disorder and rates of service utilization. *Archives of General Psychiatry, 44,* 832–836.

P. 136, *Pseudoneurological symptoms may be especially predictive of later functional disability:* Campo, J. V., & Fritsch, S. L. (1994). *ibid.*

P. 136, *Chronic fatigue syndrome appears to be a nonprogressive disease:* Dale, J. K., & Straus, S. E. (1992). *ibid.*

P. 137, *Adoption studies have shown:* Bohman, M., Cloninger, C. R., von Knorring, A.-L., & Sigvardsson, S. (1984). An adoption study of somatoform disorders: III. Cross-fostering analysis and genetic relationship to alcoholism and criminality. *Archives of General Psychiatry, 41,* 872–878; Cloninger, C. R., Sigvardsson, S., von Knorring, A.-L., & Bohman, M. (1984). An adoption study of somatoform disorders: II. Identification of two discrete somatoform disorders. *Archives of General Psychiatry, 41,* 863–871.

P. 137, *Studies have also found evidence . . . Attention Deficit Hyperactivity Disorder (ADHD):* Morrison, J. R., & Stewart, M. A. (1973). The psychiatric status of the legal families of adopted hyperactive children. *Archives of General Psychiatry, 28,* 888–891.

P. 137, *Having a male or female relative with antisocial personality increases the risk for development of Somatization Disorder:* American Psychiatric Association. (1994). *ibid.*

P. 137, *A "hysterical" informational-processing pattern:* Cloninger, C. R. (1994). *ibid.*

P. 137, *Somatic symptoms have been referred to as "body language" for emotional expression:* Nemzer, E. D. (1991). Somatoform disorders. In M. Lewis (Ed.), *Child and adolescent psychiatry: A comprehensive textbook.* Baltimore: Williams & Wilkins, p. 701.

P. 137, *chronic fatigue syndrome is characterized by the onset of persistent or relapsing debilitating fatigue:* Dale, J. K., & Straus, S. E. (1992). *ibid.*

P. 140, *In DSM-IV, pain of sufficient severity to warrant clinical attention is the primary criteria for Pain Disorder:* American Psychiatric Association. (1994). *ibid.,* pp. 458–462.

P. 140, *Headaches, recurrent abdominal pain, limb pain, and chest pain . . . 7 to 30 percent:* Campo, J. V., & Fritsch, S. L. (1994). *ibid.*

P. 141, *The symptom of pain can serve the unconscious goal of removing the individual from a conflictual situation:* Ramsay, A. R. (1984). *ibid;* Stinnett, J. L. (1987). *ibid.*

P. 141, *a "pain-prone patient or disorder":* Engel, G. L. (1959). Psychogenic pain and the pain-prone patient. *American Journal of Medicine, 26,* 899–918;

Roy, R. (1985). Engel's pain-prone disorder patient: 25 years after. *Psychotherapeutics and Psychosomatics, 43,* 126–135.

P. 141, *Studies have shown that the concentrations of serotonin and endorphin metabolites:* Cloninger, C. R. (1994). *ibid;* Kaufman, D. M. (1990). *Clinical neurology for psychiatrists* (3rd ed.). Philadelphia: Saunders.

P. 141, *a "vicious cycle of progressive deterioration":* Cloninger, C. R. (1994). *ibid.,* p. 187.

P. 142, *Conversely, health-related behaviors will diminish, as they are no longer subject to systematic reinforcement:* Cloninger, C. R. (1994). *ibid;* Fordyce, W. E., Fowler, R. S., Lehmann, J. F., DeLateur, B. J., Sand, P. L., & Trieschmann, R. B. (1973). Operant conditioning in the treatment of chronic pain. *Archives of Physical Medicine & Rehabilitation, 54,* 399–408.

P. 142, *The following factors within a family have been found to be associated with these disorders:* Jamison, R. N., & Walker, L. S. (1992). Illness behavior in children of chronic pain patients. *International Journal of Psychiatry in Medicine, 22,* 329–342; Mohamad, S. N., Weisz, G. M., & Waring, E. M. (1978). The relationship of chronic pain to depression, marital adjustment, and family dynamics. *Pain, 5,* 285–292.

P. 142, *Minuchin described four specific family transactional patterns that can relate to pain disorders:* Minuchin, S., Baker, L., Rosman, B. L., Liebman, R., Milman, L., & Todd, T. C. (1975). *ibid.*

P. 142, *Studies investigating the effects of ethnicity:* Cloninger, C. R. (1994). *ibid.*

P. 143, *etiologic to the pain syndrome:* Mufson, M. J. (1994). Chronic pain syndrome: Integrating the medical and psychiatric evaluation and treatment. In W. T. Branch (Ed.), *Office practice of medicine* (3rd ed., pp. 1019–1027). Philadelphia: Saunders.

P. 143, *You should obtain the history of prior episodes of pain in the patient:* Mufson, M. J., & McGrath, P. J. (1995). Annotation: Aspects of pain in children and adolescents. *Journal of Child Psychology and Psychiatry, 36,* 717–730; Jellinek, M. S., & Herzog, D. B. (1991). Introduction to psychiatric consultation with children. In N. H. Cassem (Ed.), *Massachusetts General Hospital handbook of general psychiatry* (3rd ed., pp. 491–507). St. Louis: Mosby-Year Book.

P. 143, *Infrared thermography may be helpful in identifying changes in temperature and vascular flow:* Cloninger, C. R. (1994). *ibid.*

P. 143, *The Minnesota Multiphasic Personality Inventory (MMPI):* Butcher, J. N., Williams, C. L., Graham, J. R., Telegen, A., & Kaemmer, B. (1992). *Minnesota Multiphasic Personality Inventory—Adolescent: Manual for administration, scoring, and interpretation.* Minneapolis: University of Minnesota Press.

P. 143, *The Personality Inventory for Children:* Pritchard, C. T., Ball, J. D., & Culbert, J. (1988). Using the Personality Inventory for Children to identify children with somatoform disorders: MMPI findings revisited. *Journal of Pediatric Psychology, 13,* 237–245.

P. 144, *Lesse coined the term* masked depression: Lesse, S. (1974). Atypical facial pain of psychogenic origin: The masked depressive syndrome. In S. Lesse (Ed.), *Masked depression.* New York: Aronson.

P. 144, *The potential demoralization and learned helplessness:* Ramsay, A. R. (1984). *ibid;* Rubin, E. H., Zorumski, C. F., & Guze, S. B. (1986). Somatoform disorders. In T. Millo & G. L. Klerman (Eds.), *Contemporary directions in psychopathology: Toward the DSM-IV* (pp. 520–533). New York: Guilford Press; Davidson, J., Krishnan, R., & France, R. (1985). Neurovegetative symptoms in chronic pain and depression. *Journal of Affective Disorders, 9,* 213–218.

P. 144, *This disorder is generally described in adults:* Schreier, H. A., & Libow, J. A. (1993). *ibid.*

P. 144, *Factitious Disorder by Proxy:* American Psychiatric Association. (1994). *ibid;* Schreier, H. A., & Libow, J. A. (1993). *ibid.*

P. 144, *This syndrome most often presents with preschool children as the patient:* Rosenberg, D. A. (1987). *ibid.*

P. 145, *Follow-up studies with patients with recurrent abdominal pain found that 25 to 50 percent:* Campo, J. V., & Fritsch, S. L. (1994). *ibid.*

P. 145, *Somatization describes a process in which a child and family seek medical help:* Murphy, M. R. (1989). Somatization: Embodying the problem. *British Medical Journal, 298,* 1331–1332.

P. 145, *Unexplained physical symptoms are common and problematic in many pediatric practices:* Campo, J. V., & Fritsch, S. L. (1994). *ibid.*

6

PAIN AND RELATED PROBLEMS

Julie A. Collier

RANDY

Randy was seven years old when he had his second heart surgery. I was asked by the surgeon to see him on the second postoperative day because he was refusing to eat or ambulate. The surgeon was concerned that this child had a "behavior problem." When I entered the room I observed a very sullen child lying in bed, with his mother hovering anxiously over him.

After a few minutes of introductions and explanations about my role, I asked Randy if he was having any pain. As he nodded his head, his eyes began to fill with tears. He told me he had been having a lot of pain and was afraid to move because "it might hurt more." His anxiety about current pain was being exacerbated by concerns about a future heart surgery he would need and the pain he was likely to experience then.

A review of the medical chart revealed that the surgeon had written an order for pain medication "PRN" (as necessary). Randy had not routinely asked for pain medication because he wanted to "act big," and he had not been routinely asked by medical staff about his level of discomfort. His parents were not aware that they could advocate for more aggressive pain management on Randy's behalf.

In my position as a psychologist in a pediatric hospital, I see many children like Randy whose encounter with a painful condition overwhelms their ability to cope effectively. It has been estimated that 35 percent of children have a chronic condition. For many of these children, pain is an unwelcome fact of life. An even greater number of children unaffected by chronic conditions will experience significant pain related to brief illnesses, surgery, or traumatic injury. Because poorly managed pain can exert a deleterious impact on a child's physical and emotional development and adaptation, it represents an important mental health issue.

In this chapter I discuss the nature of pediatric pain and review the factors that influence pain perception and behavior in the school-age child. This will be followed by a discussion of issues related to the assessment and treatment of pediatric pain.

Entire books have been written about pediatric pain. This chapter in no way represents a comprehensive discussion but is meant to be an introductory overview for all clinicians interested in working with children in pain or who are confronted with this issue in their daily practice.

WHAT IS PAIN?

Pain is a complex phenomenon that comprises physical, sensory, autonomic, and psychological elements. It cannot be predicted solely by the nature or extent of tissue damage because of the multitude of factors that interact to produce pain perception and the expression of pain behavior.

The International Association for the Study of Pain has defined pain as "an unpleasant sensory and emotional experience associated with actual or potential tissue damage, or described in terms of such damage." According to this definition, all pain has an emotional or psychological component, and it is this component of pain that can account for a substantial degree of variability in pain reactivity between children and in the same child at different points in time.

The factors that influence how a child perceives and responds to tissue damage include the child's age, sex, developmental level, pain history, and a variety of other contextual and psychological factors.

Patricia McGrath's model (depicted in Figure 6.1) of the situational, behavioral, and emotional factors that affect pain illustrates the range of factors that are important to consider when evaluating and treating the child in pain. In the figure, the characteristics listed in the closed box represent the relatively stable factors that influence the child's perception of pain. The situational, behavioral, and emotional factors listed at the top of the figure vary dynamically depending on the context. These context-specific factors interact and mutually influence one another. Discussion of each of these factors is beyond the scope of this chapter. However, because of the importance of cognitive developmental factors in pediatric pain, I will provide a brief overview.

Cognitive Development and Pediatric Pain

Children's ability to understand and communicate about pain appears to follow a developmental sequence that corresponds to Piaget's stages of cognitive development. The four main stages of cognitive development and their approximate corresponding ages are (1) the sensory-motor (birth to two years), (2) the preoperational (two to seven years), (3) the concrete operational (eight to ten years), and (4) the formal operational (eleven to fourteen years and older). Because this chapter's focus is pain in the school-age child, I don't include the sensory-motor stage in the following discussion.

Preoperational Stage. Children in the preoperational stage of cognitive development understand pain as a physical entity that has unpleasant and aversive qualities. Children in this stage may attribute pain to the transgression of rules, as in the case of a four-year-old boy who said that he had pain in his arm because

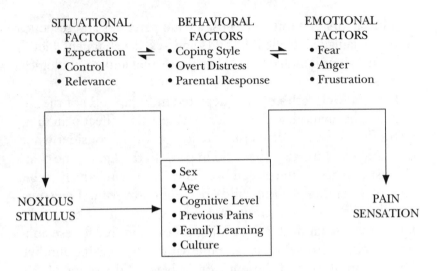

Figure 6.1
A Model of the Situational, Behavioral, and
Emotional Factors That Affect a Child's Pain

Source: Schechter, N. L., Berde, C. B., & Yaster, M. (Eds.). (1993). *Pain in infants, children and adolescents.* Baltimore: Williams & Wilkins. Reprinted by permission.

he had broken his mother's vase. It has been suggested that if a child believes that he has the pain because of some transgression, he may be less likely to complain about pain. This has implications for the treatment of pain: to rely on a child's formal complaint of pain as an indicator of whether or not he is in need of pain medication may be inadequate.

Because the thinking of the preoperational child is perceptually dominated, care should be taken to avoid exposing them to the sight of unpleasant pathology or medical instruments. Prior to the age of about six, children tend to have a passive attitude toward coping with pain. This, coupled with young children's lack of perceived control, leads to a greater dependence on others (usually parents) to assist them with coping. It is unrealistic to expect the very young child to learn to use pain-coping strategies independently. Children under the age of about seven or eight generally require a "coach."

Concrete Operational Stage. As children move into the concrete operational stage of development, their understanding of pain broadens from a focus on the purely physical aspects of pain to include an awareness of the negative affect associated with pain (for example, pain can make you sad, worried, angry, and so on). Toward the end of this stage children become aware of the variability of pain as well as the uncertainty of duration and the unpredictability of onset. A nine-year-old boy with whom I worked told me that the worst thing about his episodes of abdominal pain was that he never knew when they were going to occur. Between episodes of pain he felt "worried." During an episode of pain he felt "mad."

This expanding ability of the older school-age child to describe the qualitative and affective features of pain makes the use of suitable pediatric pain questionnaires of greater value. Although the child at this stage is capable of generating objective explanations for her pain, transgression explanations may still be present.

By the end of the concrete operational stage, pain may be viewed as dangerous, threatening, or indicative of the possibility of death. I have seen this to be particularly relevant for children with a chronic or life-threatening illness. For many of these children, each new pain, or the intensification of an existing pain, is perceived to be synonymous with progression of their disease.

Unlike the passive stance toward pain characteristic of the preoperational child, the concrete operational child now views more active physical strategies (for example, rubbing the sore area or exercising) as useful. As children progress through this stage they become increasingly capable of using behavioral pain-coping strategies independently.

Formal Operations Stage. During the stage of formal operations, children acquire the capacity to think about pain in more abstract and less perceptually dominated ways. The adolescent can appreciate the biological usefulness of pain, and she puts more emphasis on the psychological aspects of pain. Adolescents are more able to understand the value of psychological, behavioral, and cognitive techniques for reducing pain.

When discussing stages of cognitive development, we need to keep in mind that severe stress can result in regression, so that a child may exhibit thinking that is characteristic of a younger child. It is also possible for experience with illness to lead to more mature concepts of illness and pain.

Types of Pain

The types of pain children experience can be divided into three categories: acute, recurrent, and chronic.

Acute Pain. All children experience episodes of acute pain, ranging from bumps and scrapes to sprains or broken bones. Other sources of acute pain include invasive medical or dental procedures such as surgery, lumbar punctures, bone marrow aspirates, injections, or tooth extractions. Acute pain is relatively brief in duration, but when severe can exert a profound impact on a child's emotional status. This was exemplified by Randy, the boy with postoperative pain described at the beginning of this chapter.

Recurrent Pain. Recurrent pain is pain that exists in the absence of a well-defined or specific disease state. Case examples of recurrent pain syndromes include eight-year-old Carl, who missed an average of three days of school a month because of severe headaches; ten-year-old Lisa, who had repeated visits to her pediatrician for unexplained abdominal pain; and five-year-old Timmy, who frequently woke up crying during the night complaining of pain in his legs (diagnosed as growing pain). Pain episodes such as migraine and tension headaches, recurrent abdominal pain, or recurrent limb pain are often triggered by stress, and children usually function normally and are pain-free between episodes.

Chronic Pain. Children are identified as having chronic pain if their pain persists for a prolonged period of time or persists after injuries have apparently healed. Disease or injury is usually the cause of chronic pain. For children like nine-year-old Edward, chronic disease is the cause of their pain. Edward, who had juvenile rheumatoid arthritis, experienced swelling and stiffness in several joints, including his knees and ankles. On the days when his pain was particularly severe, he required a wheelchair. Other chronic illnesses that are commonly associated with pain include sickle cell anemia and hemophilia. The pain and physical debilitation that is often associated with these types of diseases can make psychological adjustment very difficult.

Surgery and traumatic injuries such as burns or fractures can cause chronic pain. Often, the chronicity of the pain is related to the severity of tissue damage, which prolongs the period of healing. Sometimes an injury is associated with nerve damage. In these cases, the pain may persist long after the apparent healing period. This was the case for Ray, an eleven-year-old boy who broke both wrists in a baseball accident and who continued to have burning pain following removal of the arm casts. He was diagnosed with a condition called reflex sympathetic dystrophy.

ASSESSING PEDIATRIC PAIN

An objective and thorough assessment of the child's pain and the related situational and psychological factors is essential for accurate medical diagnosis and effective intervention. However, the objective assessment of pain in children can be a challenge for both parents and clinicians because of a variety of cognitive and developmental factors that influence a child's response to pain as well as her ability to express the qualitative aspects of pain.

Children's pain can be assessed by a variety of behavioral, physiological, or psychological measures. There are two structured interviews developed recently that are valuable tools for the assessment of the child with recurrent or chronic pain. The first is the Varni/Thompson Pediatric Pain Questionnaire (VTPPQ), which is completed independently by the child and parent. It provides information about the sensory, affective, and evaluative dimensions of the child's pain through the use of color-coded rating scales, visual analog scales, and verbal descriptors. It also provides information about the child's and family's pain histories, pain relief interventions, and social and environmental situations that may influence the pain. The VTPPQ was initially evaluated using a sample of twenty-five children (four to nineteen years old) with juvenile rheumatoid arthritis.

The Children's Comprehensive Pain Questionnaire (CCPQ), developed by Patricia McGrath, also uses a variety of rating scales and interview questions to assess multiple dimensions of a child's recurrent or chronic pain. The CCPQ has been used with three hundred children (ages five to sixteen), with good initial validity and reliability. McGrath has also developed an interview measure for assessment of acute and procedural pain that follows a similar format.

MANAGING PEDIATRIC PAIN

Because of the central role of psychological factors in pain, you have a great deal to offer children experiencing pain. In order for your treatment to be most effective, you need to have an adequate understanding of the range of pain management techniques available.

Distraction

Distraction is one of the most commonly employed pain management techniques. Although distraction has been perceived as merely a simple diversionary tactic in which the child attends to something other than the presence of pain, recent animal research has suggested that distraction may have a more complex function. The animal studies demonstrated that neuronal activity evoked by a constant noxious stimulus varied depending on the animal's attention. Thus, the use of distraction may actually reduce a child's response to an unpleasant stimulus at a neuronal level.

Central to the effectiveness of distraction techniques is the child's ability to attend fully to something other than his pain. Some of the most commonly used distraction strategies include watching TV, playing video games, singing, squeezing someone's hand, describing a favorite place, or describing a novel object. Many of the other pain management techniques, such as relaxation, hypnosis, music, and so on, also involve a component of distraction. Obviously, because the effectiveness of distraction depends on the child's ability to concentrate fully on something, the choice of strategy is key and must be something that appeals to and easily engages the child.

Relaxation and Imagery

Relaxation interventions are commonly used to treat anxiety and pain in children. The exact mechanisms by which relaxation produces pain relief are not well understood. Proposed mechanisms include decreases in ischemic pain as a result of a reduction of muscle tension, changes in brain chemistry (particularly serotonin metabolism), increased feelings of control, a reduction of autonomic reactivity, and distraction.

There are many approaches to relaxation, and the techniques of biofeedback, guided imagery, hypnosis, and music therapy all facilitate physical and mental relaxation. I frequently use a deep breathing exercise in which the child is taught to breathe deeply, noticing that with each exhalation, his body becomes a bit more calm and relaxed. The slower and deeper the breathing, the more his body relaxes.

I also frequently use progressive muscle relaxation in which the child is taught to tighten and relax different muscle groups. A variety of helpful scripts have been published for teaching children progressive muscle relaxation. I often incorporate imagery to facilitate relaxation. Imagery can also make the experience more fun and enjoyable for children.

Biofeedback

The technique of biofeedback involves amplifying and translating the body's nonobservable electrical activity into observable auditory or visual signals. It is an excellent tool for teaching relaxation because it provides direct and immediate feedback about bodily states, helping the child learn to distinguish between relaxed and tense conditions. It has been most commonly used to treat pediatric tension and migraine headaches but can be helpful for a variety of pain problems.

Hypnosis

Hypnosis is another commonly used pain management technique. The mechanisms underlying the effectiveness of hypnosis are not well understood. One theory is that hypnosis represents an altered state of consciousness, or trance state, during which an individual is highly susceptible to suggestions.

There is a great deal of individual variability in hypnotic responsiveness, and children tend to demonstrate greater hypnotic susceptibility than adults. Standardized hypnotic susceptibility tests suggest that children's hypnotic susceptibility rises rapidly at around age four or five and reaches a maximum at around eight to twelve years of age. Scores then gradually decrease with age, although some individuals maintain a high level of hypnotic susceptibility throughout their lives.

Music Therapy

Music therapy has been documented to have beneficial physical and psychological effects for individuals in pain, and can be a simple and useful adjuvant to many other pain management techniques. Children can be encouraged to choose musical recordings that will help them focus their attention away from their pain. It can be a particularly helpful aid in cases where children have trouble falling asleep because of their pain.

Thought-Stopping

In its original form, thought-stopping was one of the early behavior modification techniques. Dorothea Ross developed a modification of this strategy for children experiencing anticipatory anxiety prior to painful procedures or other aversive events. The child is helped to identify a list of positive facts about the impending procedure. ("It doesn't take long. It will help me get better. I get a sticker when I'm done.") She is then helped to think of some reassuring facts. ("If I use my distraction techniques, it won't hurt as much. When it's over I won't have to worry about it for a whole month.") The facts are condensed so that the child can easily memorize the material. She is instructed that whenever she thinks about the impending painful procedure, she must stop what she is doing and recite the entire set of sentences, subvocally if others are in the room, or aloud if she is alone. This procedure helps to eliminate the feeling of helplessness in the face of an aversive event, providing the child with a greater sense of control.

Operant Techniques

The operant techniques are based on the principles of operant conditioning. In this model, behavior is governed by its consequences. Behavior that leads to a positive outcome will be maintained or will increase; behavior that is followed by a negative outcome will decrease.

In some pediatric pain cases, the child's pain complaints elicit overly solicitous responses from his parents. He may receive extra attention, and the usual demands and expectations may be reduced. The pain behavior is reinforced and is therefore much more likely to continue or increase. In cases such as this, parents must be helped to shift their focus from "ill" behavior to adaptive behavior; they need to respond positively to adaptive attempts to cope with pain and to other nonpain behaviors. Examples of techniques based on operant principles include reinforcement (for example, praising the child's attempt to use relaxation to manage his pain); extinction (ignoring the child's maladaptive pain behaviors); and shaping (gradually increasing the criteria for rewards).

Modeling

Modeling, or observational learning, is another useful technique. Children can be helped to manage their fears and cope more effectively by observing a model or peer who copes effectively with a similar type of pain. There are a few videos that aim to prepare children for hospitalization, surgery, or painful procedures by depicting a child model coping successfully with the experience.

I find the use of a model particularly helpful when working with a child who is fearful of medical procedures, and I will often ask a child who has learned to cope well with a procedure if she would be willing to demonstrate her skills to another patient. Most children are quite proud of their newfound pain-coping skills and will readily display their talents.

Desensitization

Systematic desensitization refers to a process of gradual exposure to an anxiety-provoking object or situation in a progressive sequence, leading to an eventual reduction of anxiety. Exposure to the feared stimulus is paired with the incompatible response of relaxation. This technique is most useful for conditioned anxiety and fear associated with painful medical procedures. You first identify the anxiety-provoking aspects of the process, impart the relaxation skills, and then gradually expose the child to the feared stimuli in practice sessions.

Art Therapy, Play Therapy, and Psychotherapy

Art and play are the natural medium for children to express themselves. Both art and play can facilitate assessment of a child's emotional state as well as offer a means of expressing distress and working through conflicts.

Some patients require a more in-depth psychotherapeutic approach. In cases where a patient's symptoms do not appear to be responsive to the standard cognitive-behavioral techniques or if a patient appears unmotivated to learn more adaptive ways to manage his pain, a more traditional psychotherapeutic approach may be indicated. Often, it is only after exploration and resolution of the meaning of pain and the role it plays in his family that a patient can begin to engage in more productive attempts to manage his pain.

Choice of Techniques

When reviewing this list of techniques, a logical question is, "Which technique(s) do I use?" There are no well-defined criteria for selecting a method. Often, the particular techniques chosen reflect the bias of the therapist; one therapist may have a preference for progressive muscle relaxation, whereas another prefers to use guided imagery to promote a relaxed state.

For many therapists, unfortunately, the type of pain often influences the choice of technique. Certain pain management techniques have become matched to certain types of pain, without attention to the relevant situational, familial, or emotional factors that contribute to the pain of a particular patient. For example, a child with recurrent headaches may be referred directly to a biofeedback specialist, without a full assessment of the contextual factors related to the pain.

This was the case with ten-year-old Maggie, who was referred to me following a failed attempt at biofeedback for her headaches. My assessment suggested that her complaints of headaches were complicated by symptoms of separation anxiety. Complaints of headache pain increased in the face of impending separations from her mother. Eventually, Maggie did benefit from biofeedback, but only after the relevant contextual issue (difficulty with separation) was addressed.

As suggested in Maggie's case, the choice and timing of intervention techniques are largely driven by the case formulation. To arrive at the formulation, you must consider the effect of each realm of influence depicted in McGrath's model of the situational, behavioral, and emotional factors that affect a child's pain (Figure 6.1). Let's look at two cases that were referred to me for management of distress during painful procedures.

JENNY

Nine-year-old Jenny was very anxious during procedures. Her parents were attentive and nurturing, but they were not sure how to help their daughter. Intervention was relatively straightforward with this family. I taught Jenny two relaxation strategies, one using breathing and the other using imagery. I demonstrated them for her parents and discussed how the parents could support her during procedures. Jenny's distress was significantly reduced one month later.

JEFFREY

Eight-year-old Jeffrey was beginning his second course of treatment following a relapse of his leukemia. Although he had managed procedures fairly well during his first treatment, he had been reacting very intensely to procedures since the relapse. His parents were understandably distraught, and they became extremely anxious themselves during procedures. This, in turn, exacerbated Jeffrey's anxiety.

I taught Jeffrey a number of relaxation and distraction strategies that he was to use before and during procedures. However, unlike in Jenny's case, I needed to draw on additional intervention strategies. I incorporated operant techniques with the parents, who were instructed to praise positive coping behaviors rather than react intensely to expressions of distress. I also incorporated play and art therapy in order to give Jeffrey additional avenues to express his anger about the relapse. Over the course of the next several weeks, Jeffrey began to cope more effectively with his treatment.

These cases illustrate that, despite the same referral problem—management of distress during painful procedures—the constellation of mediating factors dictated the selection of different techniques.

Also included in the case formulation are any individual characteristics of the child that lend themselves to one technique over another. For example, the ability to create imagery varies from person to person. Some individuals are capable of experiencing very vivid images, whereas others find it very difficult to conjure a clear image upon request. Obviously, you do not want to rely on the technique of guided imagery if your patient has a limited capacity for imagery. Instead, you may wish to use something like progressive muscle relaxation.

It is also important to take into account the interests, hobbies, and preferences of the child. This may influence, for example, the type of imagery used. Some children prefer mountain scenes over beaches, or images of activity (such as a baseball game or rides at Disneyland) over images of tranquility. Some prefer sensations of warmth; others prefer sensations of coolness. I try to incorporate favorite hobbies when possible. For example, one child with whom I worked loved computers. I had him imagine that he could see the outline of his body on a computer screen, with the painful areas lit up in red (the color he chose to represent pain). I then had him imagine that he was typing information into the computer that resulted in the red areas gradually changing to blue (the color he associated with physical comfort).

Because there is no clear template for choice of technique, you may start with one technique and then find that it must be modified or that another approach is indicated. For example, I began by using progressive muscle relaxation with one of my patients. After a couple of sessions, he admitted that he found the process "boring," which also meant it was not very relaxing. I then switched to a guided imagery approach, using images of magic carpet rides and spaceship voyages. The change in strategy was made in the context of our therapeutic "partnership" to explore and discover what strategies would work best for him.

In another case, a child had difficulty learning to use relaxation strategies because of a limited awareness of changes in his body. He did much better with biofeedback because of the concrete "feedback" he received about the changes he achieved through the use of relaxation. Both of these cases underscore the importance of carefully monitoring a patient's progress in order to judge the effectiveness of the techniques you have chosen.

Pharmacological Pain Management

It is important for the mental health clinician working in the area of pediatric pain to be very familiar with the variety of pharmacological pain management interventions available. In most cases of pediatric pain, psychological or nonpharmacological techniques will be used in conjunction with some type of medication regimen, particularly in cases of moderate to severe pain.

Multidisciplinary Collaboration

Because most patients will benefit from a combination of interventions that span several professional domains, including those of medicine, nursing, physical therapy, and psychology, multidisciplinary collaboration is essential in the management of pediatric pain. For the practitioner in private practice, this may mean frequent phone contact with a child's pediatrician in order to coordinate care and remain mutually informed of a patient's progress.

For clinicians whose primary work setting is a pediatric hospital, collaboration among disciplines may come in the form of a multidisciplinary pain team or clinic. At Lucile Salter Packard Children's Hospital at Stanford, our pain team consists of an anesthesiologist, a clinical nurse specialist, a physical therapist, and a psychologist, with involvement of professionals from other disciplines, such as pharmacy, occupational therapy, or art therapy, when indicated in a particular case.

Many of the pain management cases I see are referred to our pain service. However, I frequently receive requests to evaluate an adjustment or behavioral issue in pediatric patients for whom pain is not the presenting referral question. This was the case with Randy, the seven-year-old boy introduced at the beginning of this chapter. In cases such as this, it is often your role to educate the referring physician about the role that pain plays in a patient's problems.

GENERAL PRINCIPLES

Before discussing specifics about treating acute, recurrent, and chronic pain, it is helpful to review some general treatment principles that apply to all cases.

Include Parents

Including parents in the intervention process is vital. Because parents are the primary source of support for a child, they are principle players in the treatment process. Obviously, their behavior will affect the child's response during a painful episode, and this is a necessary focus of treatment. But perhaps more important, the parents must understand the nature of pain and the rationale for the interventions. If this is lacking, they will communicate to the child in direct and indirect ways their doubt about the efficacy of the interventions.

ERIC

I encountered this dynamic with nine-year-old Eric, who was hospitalized for an episode of pain related to his sickle cell anemia. I was asked by his hematologist to assist him with pain management. Prior to my involvement, a well-meaning nurse had attempted to do some guided imagery with him to help him with his pain. I was informed by Eric and his father that this intervention did little to ease his discomfort. His father went on to tell me (and had already told the nurse while in Eric's presence) that he didn't believe in that "new age stuff," referring not only to guided imagery but to most other cognitive-behavioral pain management strategies as well. Clearly this belief, now shared by Eric, was an impediment to effective intervention and needed to be incorporated as a primary treatment target.

Thus, the first step in any treatment plan is education of the patient and parents about the complex nature of pain. We emphasize the plasticity of pain and the variety of psychological and environmental factors that can influence pain perception. Children and parents should be encouraged to think of situations in which the child's perception of pain was altered; for example, she might not have felt the pain from a scrape because she was concentrating on her soccer game. The goal of this initial step is to facilitate an understanding of how modification of a variety of psychological factors through cognitive and behavioral techniques can reduce their child's experience of pain.

For Eric and his father, this was the key to further intervention. His father listened intently as I explained what we know from research on pain about the plasticity of pain and the factors that can modify pain perception. Involving the father in a discussion of clinical research enabled him to view subsequent suggestions for nonpharmacological pain management in the context of "scientific research" rather than "hocus-pocus." This set the stage for therapeutic success.

Often, the clinician will need to work with parents to modify their responses to their child's pain. For instance, during painful procedures it is common for a parent's own anxiety about the procedure or illness to exacerbate a child's level of distress. Inconsistent responses to complaints of pain can also reinforce a child's overt distress, particularly in cases of recurrent or chronic pain. In these cases, parents may vary their responses, either providing excessive emotional and physical support or indicating that they do not have the time to assist their child. The child receives the message that his complaints of pain must be stronger to convince his parents that he needs the same degree of support that he received in the past. Obviously, including the parents in the treatment process is essential, and may involve intervention at a number of levels—from teaching them skills to help their child cope, to modifying their responses to their child's physical and emotional distress.

Offer Options

All children should be taught several interventions so they can develop a flexible repertoire of pain-coping strategies. It is unlikely that the same strategy will be useful with each episode or with each type of pain.

For example, one of my patients, who had bone cancer, usually relied on the use of imagery to cope with episodes of pain. However, occasionally she felt too tired or overwhelmed by other factors to concentrate on her imagery effectively. When this occurred, she resorted to the use of breathing techniques that helped keep her calm and distracted during the pain. Knowing that she had more than one strategy for managing her pain helped her feel a greater sense of control and mastery in the face of an inherently unpredictable situation.

Prepare for "Paradoxical" Responses to Treatment

Some children may report that their experience of pain actually increases for a short time following the initiation of treatment. This is particularly true for children who have been denying or avoiding the experience of emotional distress, as we see in the next case.

VICKY

Ten-year-old Vicky had recurrent headaches. She denied experiencing any distress about a number of stressors in her life, yet her symptom diary revealed that the frequency of her headaches increased during times of stress. As we began to explore the relationship between stress and pain, Vicky began to talk about the distress she had been internalizing. Her reports of headache pain increased during the first two weeks of treatment but then began to decline steadily as she developed new skills for managing stress and difficult emotions.

The occurrence of an increase in pain following the initiation of intervention that is expected to relieve pain can be upsetting for children and their parents, and can lead to premature termination of treatment. Adequate preparation and education prior to the initiation of treatment can prevent undue frustration for families. In Vicky's case, I predicted for the family that Vicky was likely to experience a brief exacerbation of her headaches, and assured them that it would only be temporary and that it was actually a good sign that we were on the right track in helping Vicky identify troubling emotional issues.

Teach the Importance of Practice

Finally, it is important to convey to children and their parents that the pain management techniques they will learn require practice. It is unlikely that after only one session they will learn to use a particular technique with significant success.

The treatment process is about developing new skills. The development of any new skill takes practice. I often use the metaphor of learning to ride a bike. When a child learns to ride a bike, she starts out feeling awkward and unsteady, often requiring the assistance of training wheels. With practice, she develops better balance, eventually enough to have the training wheels removed. In time, the skill of riding a bike becomes so automatic that she doesn't even think about it anymore. She just gets on and rides. And so it is with pain management: with practice, she will automatically know what to do to reduce discomfort.

MANAGING ACUTE PAIN

All children will experience a variety of acute pains during childhood, from minor injuries or illnesses to routine immunizations. Some unfortunate children, however, experience severe episodes of acute pain as a result of serious injury or painful medical procedures. During these situations, fear, anxiety, and feelings of loss of control can exacerbate a child's pain perception and behavior. Intervention for acute pain should entail a multistrategy approach, focusing on modification of situational and emotional factors. The next case example illustrates this multistrategy approach as I applied it to Peter's procedural pain.

PETER

Peter was ten years old when he was diagnosed with leukemia. He was referred to me because he was having difficulty tolerating leg injections that were a part of his treatment. With ample sedation he was able to "tolerate" bone marrow aspirations and lumbar punctures (although he still had difficulty sleeping the night before these procedures). However, the oncologist was not comfortable providing sedating medication for a simple leg shot.

On the days that Peter was to receive these shots, he would engage in a variety of stall tactics (such as requesting drinks of water, suggesting he would do better with a different nurse, negotiating how much time he needed to get himself ready). When the time arrived to receive the shot, he would begin to protest loudly, cry, and occasionally resist physically, requiring that his parents and the staff physically restrain him. The amount of time that the entire process took varied significantly, depending on which staff were working that day (and how tolerant they were).

Prior to being diagnosed with leukemia Peter had been an active, healthy child. He described the process of being treated for leukemia as "the scariest thing ever." Anxiety about the unpredictable nature of the situation and feelings of loss of control pervaded the initial interview with Peter and his parents. Peter had difficulty with all procedures but was less behaviorally resistant when given premedication. His parents were very distressed by his behavioral outbursts when he was to receive injections. They felt very guilty about participating in physical restraint of their son but did not know what else to do to help him.

Peter and his parents were eager to learn new coping strategies. They were educated about the role that situational and emotional factors play in exacerbating procedural pain. I asked Peter how long the "hurt" from the injection lasted. "Only a few seconds," he said.

I discussed the use of distraction as a coping strategy. Borrowing from Ross and Ross, I told them that our attention is a finite resource; attention to one activity limits the amount of attention we have for another activity. I used a number of examples to illustrate this point.

"What happens if you are talking on the phone to a friend, and your mom comes in the room and begins talking to you? Can you listen to everything that both people are saying to you? Of course not. You have to decide which person you are going to listen to and tell the other that he or she will have to wait a minute." I underscored the fact that Peter was in charge of a scarce resource (attention) that he could choose to allocate in any way he choose.

I went on to explain that we are much more aware of feelings and sensations if we give them all of our attention. Together, Peter and I came up with examples of this, such as being so interested in playing with friends that he didn't realize that it was past his dinnertime.

Once he stopped playing, he realized how hungry he was, a sensation he had not previously been attending to. Peter also described the experience of being hit with a baseball during an exciting game, only noticing the tenderness after the game was over.

I told Peter that I would teach him some ways to keep his attention away from the experience of discomfort during injections and that we would work together to identify several different strategies that he could choose from, because he might find that one strategy works well on some days but not on others. His parents were very involved in this process in their role as Peter's "coaches" during procedures.

Peter and I developed a list of strategies and created a chart.

Things I Can Do to Make Shots Easier

- *Squeeze Mom or Dad's hand* to tell them how much it hurts.
- *Use distraction:* focus on my breathing and blowing the scary feelings away; count backward from twenty during the shot; sing a song with Mom or Dad
- *Stay happy,* because how I feel influences how much it hurts.

I educated the nursing staff about the need to maximize predictability and control for Peter. Peter was given the choice of preparing the injection site with alcohol, adding to his sense of control. We defined in detail the procedure for injections, and the staff were encouraged to adhere to this procedure each time.

When it was time for the injection, Peter and the nurse would check the clock. Peter had a maximum of thirty minutes in which he could prepare himself and complete the injection process. If after thirty minutes he had not allowed the nurse to give the injection, the nurses were allowed to restrain him. Defining the parameters of this process meant that Peter knew exactly what would happen. The process before this time had been very erratic. Some nurses gave him little time to prepare before initiating physical restraint; others would allow the process to drag on for an hour.

In order to further facilitate Peter's adaptation to his treatment, I incorporated medical play, drawing, and peer modeling. Young children, in particular, benefit greatly from therapeutic play involving dolls or stuffed animals and the medical items used during their procedures. Peter jumped at the suggestion that he might have an opportunity to "check out" the procedure items. He was old enough to handle the type of syringe and needle used for his shots, and he took advantage of the opportunity to practice administering shots to a stuffed monkey.

Capitalizing on Peter's love of drawing, I asked him to draw pictures depicting the worst part of having leukemia and to draw pictures of himself during procedures before and after our work together. I also introduced Peter to Amelia, an eleven-year-old girl with whom I had previously worked. Amelia described her favorite coping strategies and allowed Peter to watch her cope successfully during a blood draw.

The initial skills instruction consisted of three sessions over the course of two weeks, after which Peter was able to cooperate consistently within the thirty-minute time frame, without the use of physical restraint. The drawing, medical play, and peer modeling took place during sessions four through six. At this point Peter was able to complete the injection process within five minutes. The focus of the seventh and final session was on generalization of his skills to other procedures, such as bone marrow aspirates and lumbar punctures.

MANAGING RECURRENT AND CHRONIC PAIN

Recurrent pain syndromes, such as headaches, limb pain (growing pain), or abdominal pain, constitute a significant health problem. It has been estimated that as many as 33 percent of children experience recurrent abdominal pain, and 40 to 60 percent of children experience headaches. The incidence of limb or growing pain has been somewhat more difficult to establish, with estimates ranging from 4 to 18 percent of children. The inability to cope with stress is a common feature of recurrent pain syndromes and is usually a major focus of the treatment.

Chronic pain, defined as any pain that persists for a prolonged period or that persists after injuries have apparently healed, can have a major impact on psychological adjustment. Treatment must address not only the specifics of coping with the pain itself but also the depression, anxiety, social isolation, and increased dependence that occur as a result of the chronic pain.

You can use similar techniques for the treatment of both recurrent and chronic pain. Of utmost importance, however, is to ensure that your case formulation synthesizes the dynamics and issues relevant for that particular patient. The following two case examples illustrate the treatment of Aaron's recurrent pain and Emily's chronic pain.

AARON

Aaron was referred to me by his gastroenterologist for management of recurrent abdominal pain. Aaron described his pain as "stabbing like a knife." His pain was sometimes accompanied by diarrhea. At the time of the referral, he had been experiencing episodes of pain lasting thirty minutes to "several hours" approximately one time per week over the previous two months. His history revealed that he had had similar abdominal pain at the age of six. At that time the gastroenterologist recommended that Aaron increase his fiber intake and prescribed an antispasmodic medication. The pain resolved after four months.

The assessment revealed a number of psychological, behavioral, and situational factors related to Aaron's abdominal pain. Aaron was a "worrier." He worried about school performance and being accepted by peers. He was very attentive to conversations between his parents and would worry about issues they discussed, such as the family's finances. When he would begin to feel pain, he would worry that it was going to become very severe and possibly not go away.

Aaron's parents were very concerned about his abdominal pain. When Aaron experienced pain and distress, they would become distressed and anxious themselves. They would hover over him and attempt to calm him, but they inadvertently communicated their own distress to Aaron, further escalating his anxiety. They were aware that Aaron had a tendency to worry, and their strategy for managing this was to give him reasons why he should not be anxious. They also felt that encouraging him to express his anxiety would only exacerbate his distress. At the time of the assessment, Aaron's parents indicated that they were under a great deal of financial stress, and they acknowledged marital conflict.

During the first session I gave Aaron the task of keeping a pain journal in which he should record the date and time of each episode of pain, along with information about what he was doing when the pain started, what he did to manage the pain, and how long the episode lasted. I also discussed with Aaron and his parents the apparent role that anxiety played in exacerbating his pain, a point they readily agreed with. They were also open to the possibility that stress and anxiety might be associated with the onset of the painful episodes.

I began by teaching Aaron a simple progressive muscle relaxation exercise. Aaron had an active imagination and was quickly able to incorporate imagery in the form of imagining a "favorite place" that was associated with a sense of calm and relaxation. Aaron understood that he usually became very upset and "tense" when in pain, and the new relaxation techniques were going to help him "keep his body as calm as possible" during pain episodes. Aaron and I demonstrated his new skill to his parents, and I discussed the need for his parents to be available as "coaches" if Aaron needed some additional assistance relaxing himself.

I then began to work with Aaron on managing stress and anxiety in other situations, helping him to develop better coping and problem-solving skills. I also worked with his parents on modifying their response to his episodes of pain, as well as to his general anxiety. They learned to refrain from reacting with their own anxiety. Instead, they learned to calmly help Aaron generate solutions to the problem at hand and allowed him to express his distress about stressful events.

I initially worked with Aaron and his parents for ten sessions. He responded well to the interventions, and by week ten he was no longer experiencing abdominal pain. The parents contacted me three months later and asked if they could bring Aaron back to see me. They had agreed to a marital separation and were concerned about how Aaron would handle the news. In particular, they were concerned that Aaron would begin having episodes of pain again. Despite Aaron's predictable distress about the impending separation, he was able to use his anxiety management strategies effectively and did not develop further episodes of pain.

EMILY

Emily was a nine-year-old girl with juvenile rheumatoid arthritis (JRA). She was referred for nonpharmacological pain management by her rheumatologist, who was also concerned about her depressed mood. Children with JRA develop pain, stiffness, and swelling in their joints. In some cases, progressive joint deterioration leads to severely impaired mobility and increased pain.

Emily complained of "aching" pain in her wrists and ankles, and in one of her knees. Her other knee had been severely affected by an ill-advised orthopedic surgery at another medical center. She experienced a great deal of pain and stiffness in this knee, particularly in the morning. The process of getting out of bed and beginning the day caused her significant physical and emotional distress. She missed several days of school a month and was becoming increasingly isolated. She refused to participate in physical therapy because she believed that it would cause more pain.

Emily's parents were at the end of their rope. They struggled with guilt about their decision to have the knee surgery, and as a result they tended to give in to most of Emily's demands. They were concerned about Emily's depressed mood and became very distressed when Emily stated one morning that she would be "better off dead."

It was clear that chronic pain was having a profound impact on Emily's psychological adjustment to her illness and that her depressed mood was further impairing her ability to participate actively in a treatment program that would, we hoped, reduce her pain. After discussing the role of situational and psychological factors in Emily's pain, my first step was to teach Emily a simple hypnotic technique to help her gain a sense of control over her situation. In the morning, before getting out of bed, Emily focused on breathing deeply while imagining that her knee (and any other affected joints) was becoming warm and loose. With a little practice, this strategy helps ease her apprehension about getting out of bed to begin the morning routine of dressing and getting to school. She was also able to use this strategy to minimize her anxiety about engaging in physical therapy; with the help of a very sensitive physical therapist, she was able to begin making use of this treatment approach.

Once Emily was able to use a few nonpharmacological pain management strategies successfully, I turned my attention to the larger issue of her adjustment to the chronic illness. Emily made good use of the opportunity in individual therapy to express her frustration, and sometimes despair, about her illness. We examined the various ways that her illness interfered with her desired goals (making new friends, participating in school activities, and so on) and identified ways that she could "give the illness the slip" by refusing the invitation to become passive and withdrawn.

I also met with Emily's family to identify how each member had been affected by the illness, and worked with the parents to move past their guilt. This allowed them to set appropriate limits while still encouraging and supporting Emily's efforts to cope with her pain and the disruption it caused in her life.

I saw Emily and her family for a total of seventeen sessions. When we completed our work, Emily was doing well in her physical therapy. Although she continued to experience aching and stiffness in her knee, she had achieved much more joint mobility and was less impaired overall. Her school attendance improved, and she had joined the school chorus.

SOMATOFORM PAIN DISORDERS

The discussion of emotional factors thus far has focused primarily on the role of emotional reactions to pain and on recurrent pain that is influenced by maladaptive management of stress.

For some children, however, psychological factors play a more central role in the etiology or maintenance of pain.

MELISSA

Melissa was eight years old when she was admitted to the hospital for treatment of severe pain in her left foot. When she was admitted to the hospital, she was unable to bear any weight on her foot; she used crutches to walk. Melissa failed to obtain relief from several pharmacological treatments, including a trial of Lidocaine, which is a local anesthetic. At this point, her physician asked for a thorough psychological evaluation.

The evaluation revealed that Melissa's family was experiencing significant stress. Her father was an alcoholic who could be verbally harsh. Her mother was significantly depressed. Melissa tended to internalize her feelings and had great difficulty verbalizing emotional distress. The pain appeared to be a vehicle for eliciting more nurturing responses from her parents and to be related to emotional distress for which she had few outlets. As psychological treatment began to address these issues, Melissa began, with the aid of physical therapy, to bear more weight on her foot, and she eventually regained full use. She continued to complain of pain intermittently but did not become disabled by it.

Somatoform disorders, described more fully in Chapter Five, are conditions in which a patient presents with physical symptoms that cannot be fully explained by an underlying organic etiology. In these cases psychological factors appear to be linked to the symptoms.

In *DSM-IV*, a diagnosis of Pain Disorder is given when psychological factors are judged to play a significant role in the onset, severity, exacerbation, or maintenance of the pain. The symptom of pain may also be associated with a variety of other physical symptoms that may represent one of the other somatoform disorders, such as Somatization Disorder or Undifferentiated Somatoform Disorder.

In all of these disorders, the physical symptoms represent the somatic expression of psychological distress. Many of the children who present with somatoform pain problems have difficulty identifying and expressing emotion. They may overtly deny that they are upset, and in fact may appear quite calm in the face of significant stress. Reports of pain in these children are not "faked." This would imply malingering. Rather, the transduction of psychological distress into somatic complaints is an unconscious process. The child does perceive physical pain.

Making the diagnosis of somatoform or "psychogenic" pain is often difficult; it requires active and ongoing collaboration with the child's physician. There is the risk that a child's pain will be prematurely diagnosed as "psychogenic" when there is in fact an undetermined organic origin.

The diagnosis should not be based solely on negative evidence of an organic etiology but should require the presence of positive psychological evidence. Patrick McGrath suggested that the best evidence for somatoform pain is the "time locking" of pain. The mere presence of, for example, anxiety or marital distress does not suggest that unexplained pain is psychogenic in nature. If, however, a child's pain recurs predictably before school exams and resolves once the exam is over, the origin of the pain is more clear.

The final confirmation of a somatoform or psychogenic diagnosis is the child's response to psychological treatment. If the diagnosis is correct, you should expect a predictable response to the appropriate psychological treatment. If a patient's pain remains unchanged after an adequate trial of psychotherapy, an organic reevaluation is indicated.

Treatment of somatoform pain disorders can be a considerable challenge. These children and their parents are often reluctant to accept a psychological explanation for the symptoms, and they may choose to pursue additional medical explanations.

It is important to avoid engaging in a power struggle with families over the exact nature of the pain. I often explain to families that many of the patients I see have pain that the doctors can't completely explain. This can be a very frustrating experience for children and their parents, particularly because not having a medical diagnosis means that no one can say when the pain will go away. When this is the case, it is extremely important that children learn to cope with the pain so that they are able to participate as fully as possible in school, peer, and family activities.

This type of explanation sets the stage for developing an alliance in which the initial focus is on learning cognitive and behavioral strategies to manage the pain. Eventually, children can be helped to apply these coping strategies to the other problematic areas of their life.

MANAGED CARE

Most of our practices these days are influenced by managed care issues. Mental health benefits are becoming increasingly limited, and health insurance organizations frequently "carve out" the mental health services by contracting with a separate organization whose role is to administer mental health benefits. Managed care companies usually have a list of providers who have agreed to provide services at a predetermined cost. Subscribers must choose a preferred provider from this list or risk out-of-pocket expenses for mental health services.

This structure amounts to an administrative separation of mental health and medical benefits, leading to a financial mind-body dualism that unfortunately parallels the split between the psyche and the soma that still characterizes much of modern medicine. A key way that my work in pediatric pain is affected by this issue is in my ability to accept some referrals from pediatricians. In some cases, the patient's health insurance covers medical treatment at Stanford Medical Center, but the mental health benefits have been assigned to an organization that does not have a contract with Stanford or any of the individual providers. This makes the goal of active and ongoing collaboration between the psychologist and the pediatrician—so vital in the treatment of pain—difficult to achieve.

In situations like this, your creativity and persistence can yield an optimal resolution. The Pediatric Pain Clinic at Packard Children's Hospital at Stanford informs insurance companies that each child receives a comprehensive evaluation that includes the physician, physical therapist, and psychologist. The comprehensive evaluation thus requires comprehensive authorization, as it is not feasible for a psychologist outside the clinic to participate in this evaluation. We rarely have difficulty obtaining the authorization for the initial evaluation when it is presented in this way.

Sometimes, however, receiving authorization for ongoing psychological treatment in these situations proves more challenging. Although insurance companies may be willing to authorize a one-time "out of network" evaluation, they may insist that the ongoing treatment be provided by one of their own contracted therapists. In situations such as this, the pediatrician can be an ally. It has been my experience that some insurance company medical directors are responsive to a call from a pediatrician who insists that the patient's mental health care be provided in the same institution as the medical care because the substantial overlap between the psychological and medical issues warrants close co-management.

It can also be helpful to educate insurance case reviewers about the nature of the connection between the medical and psychological issues in cases of pediatric pain. It is likely that most of the therapists on their provider list will not have expertise in pediatric pain. Sometimes if case reviewers are able to appreciate that appropriate psychological intervention is likely to result in a reduction in medical costs, they may be more responsive.

COUNTERTRANSFERENCE REACTIONS

Our training in psychological issues compels us to always consider the nature of our own reactions to our clinical work. The essence of the treatment of pediatric pain is the treatment of suffering in children. Working with a child in pain can be a power-ful emotional experience for a clinician, particularly when the source of pain may be a severe or life-threatening illness or the result of a severe physical trauma. Work with patients with somatoform pain can be long and frustrating.

Some common indications of countertransference reactions that I have either experienced or observed in other clinicians include the following:

Withdrawing from the patient

Having difficulty engaging with very sick or dying patients

Spending more time talking with nurses than with the family and patient

Missing appointments or always passing by when a patient is getting tests or in the middle of treatment

Wanting to transfer the care of a patient because you feel hopeless or helpless

Being convinced of either the medical or psychological origin of the problem

Getting drawn in by a patient

Feeling overwhelmed by the medical problems

Feeling bored by the endless repetition of complaints

Referring the patient for a medication evaluation in the mid-dle of treatment

It is important to be alert to the signs of countertransference and to seek supervision or consultation with a colleague when it is clear that your reactions are interfering with the therapeutic relationship.

The treatment of pediatric pain can be an exciting and chal-lenging professional experience. I find it to be one of the most satisfying aspects of my work with pediatric patients. Rarely do we as clinicians have such an opportunity to directly affect the

physical and emotional well-being of a child, and this can be a richly rewarding experience.

NOTES

P. 154, *35 percent of children have a chronic condition:* Newcheck, P., & Taylor, W. (1992). Childhood chronic illness: Prevalence, severity, and impact. *American Journal of Public Health, 82,* 364–371.

P. 154, *It cannot be predicted solely by the nature or extent of tissue damage:* McGrath, P. A. (1990). *Pain in children: Nature, assessment, and treatment.* New York: Guilford Press.

P. 154, *International Association for the Study of Pain:* International Association for the Study of Pain, Subcommittee on Taxonomy. (1979). Pain terms: A list with definitions and notes on usage. *Pain, 6,* 249–252.

P. 155, *McGrath's model:* McGrath, P. A. (1993). Psychological aspects of pain perception. In N. L. Schechter, C. B. Berde, & M. Yaster (Eds.), *Pain in infants, children and adolescents.* Baltimore: Williams & Wilkins.

P. 155, *Piaget's stages of cognitive development:* Piaget, J., & Inhelder, B. (1969). *The psychology of the child.* New York: Routledge.

P. 155, *Children in the preoperational stage of cognitive development understand pain as a physical entity:* Gaffney, A. (1993). Cognitive developmental aspects of pain in school-age children. In N. L. Schechter, C. B. Berde, & M. Yaster (Eds.), *Pain in infants, children, and adolescents.* Baltimore: Williams & Wilkins.

P. 156, *he may be less likely to complain about pain:* Gaffney, A. (1993). *ibid.*

P. 156, *avoid exposing them to the sight of unpleasant pathology or medical instruments:* Beales, J. G. (1983). Factors influencing the expectation of pain among patients in a children's burn unit. *Burns, 9,* 187–192.

P. 156, *This, . . . leads to a greater dependence on others . . . to assist them with coping:* Gaffney, A. (1993). *ibid;* Reissland, N. (1983). Cognitive maturity and the experience of fear and pain in the hospital. *Social Science and Medicine, 17,* 1389–1395.

P. 157, *As children move into the concrete operational stage . . . their understanding of pain broadens:* Gaffney, A. (1993). *ibid.*

P. 157, *use of suitable pediatric pain questionnaires:* Gaffney, A. (1993). *ibid.*

P. 157, *pain may be viewed as dangerous, threatening, or indicative of the possibility of death:* Schultz, N. V. (1971). How children perceive pain. *Nursing Outlook, 19,* 670–673; Gaffney, A. (1993). *ibid.*

P. 157, *The adolescent can appreciate the biological usefulness of pain:* Gaffney, A. (1993). *ibid.*

P. 158, *Recurrent pain is pain that exists . . . or specific disease state:* McGrath, P. A. (1990). *ibid.*

P. 158, *Pain episodes . . . are often triggered by stress:* McGrath, P. A. (1990). *ibid.*

P. 159, *Children are identified as having chronic pain:* McGrath, P. A. (1990). *ibid.*

P. 160, *Varni/Thompson Pediatric Pain Questionnaire:* Varni, J. W., Thompson, K. L., & Hanson, V. (1987). The Varni/Thompson pediatric pain questionnaire: 1. Chronic musculo-skeletal pain in juvenile rheumatoid arthritis. *Pain, 28,* 27–38.

P. 160, *Children's Comprehensive Pain Questionnaire:* McGrath, P. A. (1990). *ibid.*

P. 161, *animal studies demonstrated that neuronal activity evoked by a constant noxious stimulus:* McGrath, P. A. (1990). *ibid.*

P. 161, *Proposed mechanisms include decreases in ischemic pain:* McGrath, P. J., & Unruh, A. M. (1993). Psychological treatment of pain in children and adolescents. In N. L. Shechter, C. B. Berde, & M. Yaster (Eds.), *Pain in infants, children, and adolescents.* Baltimore: Williams & Wilkins.

P. 161, *A variety of helpful scripts have been published . . . muscle relaxation:* Cautela, J. R., & Groden, J. (1978). *Relaxation: A comprehensive manual for adults, children, and children with special needs.* Champaign: Research Press Company; Ollendick, T. H., & Cerny, J. A. (1981). *Clinical behavior therapy with children.* New York: Plenum Press.

P. 162, *technique of biofeedback involves amplifying and translating:* McGrath, P. A. (1990). *ibid.*

P. 162, *Standardized hypnotic susceptibility tests:* London, P., & Cooper, L. M. (1969). Norms of hypnotic susceptibility in children. *Developmental Psychology, 1,* 113–124.

P. 162, *Music therapy has been documented:* Bailey, L. M. (1986). Music therapy in pain management. *Journal of Pain and Symptom Management, 1,* 25–28.

P. 163, *Children can be encouraged to choose musical recordings . . . away from their pain:* McGrath, P. A. (1990). *ibid.*

P. 163, *Dorothea Ross developed a modification of this strategy:* Ross, D. M. (1984). Thought-stopping: A coping strategy for impending feared events. *Issues in Comprehensive Pediatric Nursing, 7,* 83–89.

P. 165, *Both art and play can facilitate assessment of a child's emotional state:* McGrath, P. A. (1990). *ibid.*

P. 165, *Certain pain management techniques have become matched to certain types of pain:* McGrath, P. A. (1990). *ibid.*

P. 168, *pharmacological pain management interventions:* Schechter, N. L., Berde, C. B., & Yaster, M. (1993). *Pain in infants, children and adolescents.* Baltimore: Williams & Wilkins.

P. 171, *The child receives the message that his complaints of pain must be stronger:* McGrath, P. A. (1990). *ibid.*

P. 171, *All children should be taught several interventions:* McGrath, P. A. (1990). *ibid;* Ross, D. M., & Ross, S. A. (1988). *Childhood pain: Current issues, research, and management.* Baltimore: Urban & Schwarzenberg.

P. 174, *Borrowing from Ross and Ross:* Ross, D. M., & Ross, S. A. (1988). *ibid.*

P. 175, *Peter and I developed a list of strategies and created a chart:* McGrath, P. A. (1990). *ibid.*

P. 176, *as many as 33 percent of children experience recurrent abdominal pain:* Apley, J., MacKeith, R., & Meadow, R. (1978). *The child and his symptoms: A comprehensive approach.* Oxford, England: Blackwell.

P. 176, *experience headaches:* Jay, G. W., & Tomasi, L. G. (1981). Pediatric headaches: A one year retrospective analysis. *Headache, 21,* 5–9.

P. 181, *In DSM-IV, a diagnosis of Pain Disorder:* American Psychiatric Association. (1994). *Diagnostic and statistical manual of mental disorders* (4th ed., pp. 458–462). Washington, DC: Author.

P. 182, *Patrick McGrath suggested:* McGrath, P. J. (1995). Annotation: Aspects of pain in children and adolescents. *Journal of Child Psychology and Psychiatry, 36*(5), 717–730.

P. 182, *If the diagnosis is correct, . . . the appropriate psychological treatment:* Collier, J. A. (1995). Chronic illness and somatization. In H. Steiner (Ed.), *Treating adolescents.* San Francisco: Jossey-Bass; Gonzalez-Heydrich, J., Kerner, J. A., & Steiner, H. (1991). Testing the psychogenic vomiting diagnosis: Four pediatric patients. *American Journal of Diseases of Children, 145,* 913–916.

P. 182, *I often explain to families . . . that the doctors can't completely explain:* Collier, J. A. (1995). *ibid.*

P. 183, *This structure amounts to an administrative separation:* Collier, J. A. (1995). *ibid.*

P. 184, *the substantial overlap between the psychological and medical issues warrants close co-management:* Collier, J. A. (1995). *ibid.*

P. 185, *Some common indications of countertransference reactions:* Collier, J. A. (1995). *ibid.*

7

CHILD ABUSE

Mary J. Sanders and Jennifer Dyer-Friedman

A M Y

Amy knelt in front of the easel in the therapy room as she drew faces depicting her multiple feelings toward her stepfather. "I put two tongues stuck out because one tongue is not mad enough," she whispered. As she spoke, her tears began to splash on her bare knees. She looked down and asked, "Where is that water coming from?" I took her to the mirror so she could see that the water was coming from her eyes.

Amy was severely and chronically physically, emotionally, and sexually abused and neglected by her mother and stepfather. Her teachers noted that Amy would come to school with the same clothes on each day; apparently she had not been cleaned or changed. The teachers became concerned and reported this to Child Protective Services (CPS). Their investigation revealed that Amy frequently was forced to sleep on the porch, not being allowed to enter the home. It was later discovered that she had also been physically tortured, sexually molested, and forced to watch as her pets were killed in front of her. Amy was removed from her home, with no plans for reunification with her parents, and placed in long-term care. Amy was in therapy for one year.

Amy's story is not unusual. The National Center on Child Abuse and Neglect collects data each year regarding the incidence of abuse. In 1993, almost three million alleged victims were reported, and one million (one-third) of the cases were found to be substantiated. The median age of the child-victim was six years and the gender distribution was 53 percent girls and 46 percent boys. Alleged perpetrators were parents (79 percent), other relatives (12 percent), non-caretakers (5 percent), and foster parents and child care workers (2 percent). Almost thirteen hundred children died as a result of maltreatment. Needless to say, much abuse goes unreported and some reported abuse is false; therefore these numbers are only estimates.

Until the 1960s, physical abuse of children was considered rare, perhaps because corporal punishment of children was more accepted culturally. In 1962, Kempe, Silverman, Steele, Droege-mueller, and Silver redescribed the battered-child syndrome. In *People* v. *Jackson*, the battered-child syndrome was affirmed in the legal arena. Sexual abuse was considered to be rare until the 1970s. In 1974, the federal government passed the Child Abuse Prevention and Treatment Act, which resulted in every state's passing laws designating persons who were to report child abuse.

The purpose of this chapter is to define the areas of reportable abuse, explore the dynamics and consequences of abuse, and to describe our approach to individual and family treatment. We also describe Munchausen by proxy (MBP), a specific form of physical and emotional abuse.

The definitions of reportable child abuse may be found in each state's penal code. In general, *physical abuse* is interpreted as any injury inflicted on a child by other than accidental means. It is important to consider cultural factors in assessing whether disciplinary acts are abusive. *Sexual abuse* is defined as a sexual act (touching or exhibition) between an adult and child or between two children when one of them is significantly older or uses coercion. *Emotional abuse* occurs when a person conveys to a child that he is worthless, unloved, or endangered. *Neglect* may be any act or omission of action harming or threatening to harm the child's health or welfare, such as when a caretaker is unable or unwilling to provide basic needs (food, clothing, shelter, medical care, or supervision) or when the caretaker willfully causes or permits the child to be placed in situations such that her health is endangered.

The law requires that mandated reporters immediately call CPS or the police when they have "reasonable suspicion" of child abuse. This occurs when "it is objectively reasonable for a person to entertain such a suspicion, based on facts that could cause a reasonable person in a like position, drawing upon his or her training and experience to suspect child abuse." Mandated reporters should guard against the misinterpretation of the child's behavior or statements that may lead to inaccurate reports of abuse. Reporters should also be aware of situations in which false allegations of abuse may be more likely to be made, such as during a divorce.

Treatment begins when the report is made. This can and should be, as much as possible, a therapeutic experience. There may be a number of crises to deal with during the investigation period: removing the child, parent, or both from the home; placing the child in a shelter or in foster care; obtaining financial resources for treatment (Victim's Witness funds); and bringing criminal charges and being involved with the court.

Dynamics of Abuse

Simply put, abuse occurs when someone more powerful does not restrain herself from aggressing against another person. Likewise, neglect occurs when the more powerful adult refrains from giving needed care to the less powerful, dependent individual. Thus the adult places her needs above those of the child. Various models have been put forth in an attempt to understand the causes or determinative factors of abusive behavior.

We base our interventions on a model developed by Jay Belsky. It is our belief that abusive behavior occurs as a result of many contributing factors, rather than any single determinative factor. The contributing factors may be any combination of (1) parenting factors—for example, the parent's personality, temperament, knowledge, and expectations; (2) child factors, such as temperament, physical health, or unwitting negative behavior; (3) the family's context—for example, financial stressors, supports, or work; and (4) the greater societal or cultural values that may perpetuate family violence. As Belsky stated, "There is no one pathway to these disturbances in parenting: rather, maltreatment seems to arise when stressors outweigh supports and risks are greater than protective factors."

This model necessitates assessing multiple areas of family and individual functioning in order to create a treatment plan. Based on the assessment findings, your treatment may address the parents' behavior as evident in the parent-child interactions, the strategies to alleviate family stressors, and the effect (if any) of family-of-origin and cultural values that may perpetuate the abusive behaviors.

TREATMENT MODEL

Our treatment approach is based on Michael White's narrative model of psychotherapy. This model is integrative in its assumptions and is thereby well suited to the complex interplay of factors that can lead to abusive behaviors. The model focuses on how individuals interact rather than on pathologizing or assigning blame to individuals. We believe this approach allows perpetrators and their families to benefit from treatment.

The narrative model is based on the idea that people's behavior is informed by self-narratives that they construct about themselves in relation to their family and to society. An abusive parent's self-narrative may include many factors and events that "invite" the parent to respond to her child in an abusive manner. Our treatment encourages the individual to challenge her dominant problem-saturated stories and to discover alternate stories.

This shift reflects her ability to escape the problem-filled stories and facilitates change to more desired behaviors.

Our work with parents focuses on exploring etiological variables that promote a "dominant story" of abuse; in other words, we explore how the abusive interaction served the needs of the parent. We help him understand the effects of his abusive behaviors on his child and to take responsibility for his behaviors. And, lastly, we identify situations in which the parent does not engage in abusive behaviors and attempt to establish how that happens, in order to develop the alternative story, one in which the abuse does not occur. Our work with children focuses on counteracting the negative effects of abuse, co-constructing a self-story of health, and rebuilding relationships in which abusive behaviors do not occur.

CONSEQUENCES OF ABUSE

The abuse of a child is an abuse of power, as the adult is always in the more powerful position. When an adult places his needs above the child's needs, the child is marginalized and objectified. The child is invited to not have needs or feelings, to feel powerless, and to not have a "self." Certainly children respond differently to abuse, but overall, the dominant story the child tends to create in response to abuse involves a lack of self. In the case of Amy, she appeared to experience such a lack of self that she was unaware of her own tears.

Short-Term Effects: Harm to the Child

The available research indicates that abuse (and variables associated with abuse) may interrupt the developmental process, sometimes producing a domino effect resulting in behavioral, emotional, and social difficulties. Generally, the possible effects of abuse on the developing child are increased anxiety, depression, low self-esteem, aggressive behaviors, cognitive and developmental delays, school difficulties, and difficulties with attachment and social interaction. Some children become delinquent or violent; others turn their aggression against themselves (for example, engaging in self-abuse), becoming depressed and suicidal. Both sexually and physically abused children may commonly experience Posttraumatic Stress Disorder (PTSD) symptoms. Moreover, the abused or neglected child may be at risk for continued abuse from others in their reactions to his delays, social difficulties, and aggressive behaviors.

Long-Term Effects: Cycle of Violence

Many authors have promoted the concept of a cycle of violence, suggesting that abused children may become violent and abusive in their own adulthood. In a landmark study, Maxfield and Widom were able to track 908 victims of abuse over a twenty-two- to twenty-six-year span in a prospective study conducted in the Midwest. They found that a significantly higher percentage of abuse victims were more likely to have been arrested for violent crimes in comparison to a matched control group. Thus they concluded that being a victim of abuse places the child at more risk for engaging in criminal and violent behavior in his adult life. By extension, therefore, a parent who was abused as a child may be at higher risk for having parenting difficulties due to his own tendencies toward violence as well as to his limited repertoire of alternative parenting strategies. This finding underlines the need to provide appropriate treatment and support to abused children and their families as an attempt to break this cycle of violence.

The Impact of Abuse

It is clear that abuse and neglect are harmful to children; however, the impact of abuse is variable. Some of the factors associated with increased distress include the following: invasiveness and degree of force, frequency, duration, number of perpetrators, and the relationship between the child and perpetrator.

Mennen found that for children six to eighteen years of age, increased severity of abuse predicted a higher level of distress when the abuser was not a father figure and a lower level of distress when the perpetrator was a father figure. Mennen concluded that these contradictory findings could be explained by the children's self-blame. It seemed that when extreme force was not employed, the children blamed themselves for not preventing the abuse. In another study, the victim's "story" of the abuse was also suggested to have a mediating effect on adult adjustment. Coffey found that the more the victim felt a sense of stigma and self-blame, the poorer her adjustment was in adulthood.

Over the past few years, researchers have found that family and sociocultural factors exert a greater influence on the child's development than do the abusive or neglectful events. It may be that family variables associated with maltreatment have a more detrimental effect on the child than the abusive events themselves. Likewise, the family's ability to become supportive and nurturing of the child may positively mediate the effects of maltreatment.

CASE MANAGEMENT AND CRISIS INTERVENTION

In this chapter, we limit our discussion to intrafamilial abuse and neglect, as this represents the major portion of the cases we identify. In the case of stranger-abuse, the victim (or the victim's family) is less likely to experience a sense of betrayal or ambivalence toward the alleged perpetrator. However, children in either situation may experience similar effects as a result of the abuse, such as fear, loss of trust, and symptoms consistent with acute trauma. In both cases, too, the families may be hesitant to accept treatment: with intrafamilial abuse, family members may be hesitant to confront each other and themselves regarding the abuse and what led up to it; with stranger abuse, the family may want to distance itself from the abusive event(s) in order to return to a sense of normalcy.

Legal Implications

There may be criminal charges of the alleged perpetrator as well as involvement with either the juvenile or family court as a result of the reported abuse. The child may need to testify in court and deal with the stressors of facing the alleged perpetrator and undergoing cross-examination. Also, the child may be removed from the home, and the family may be required to take part in a treatment plan in order to be reunified.

If the family is working toward the goal of reunification, the treatment plan must contain clear goals toward that end. This requires a clearly stated therapy plan and a means of evaluating treatment success. Optimally the evaluation of treatment success will be conducted by the treatment team (physician, therapist, CPS worker) as well as an outside evaluator.

As a therapist, you may be placed in the dual role of providing support as well as monitoring progress. You may find yourself in the position of providing the court with needed information that assists their decision making. In order to fulfill both of these roles, you must be very explicit in your explanation to the family regarding what information you will be sharing. We prefer to write up a report and go over it with the family prior to sending it to the court. If the family disagrees with what is written, we will add an addendum to the report with their input. The recommendation for reunification must be based on more than simply having parents attend therapy. A decision to reunify the family is based on the parents' ability to take responsibility for their own acts, put the child's needs above their own, and provide a safe environment for him.

Treatment Contract

After addressing the initial crises and securing a safe environment for the child, you begin to make the treatment contract with the family. This contract should include an explanation to the family about the limits of confidentiality, clarification of your responsibility regarding the provision of information to CPS or the courts, and delineation of who will attend the sessions and how often they will take place. In addition, the participants in the therapy must promise that they will not commit any further acts of abuse, and safeguards must be put into place to help them uphold their promise. The goal of this contract is to avoid miscommunication and to communicate to the family that they will be collaborators in the therapy process.

Managed Care

Of increased concern is how to provide needed evaluations and treatment in a time of limited resources. In our experience, managed care companies have acknowledged the increased insurance costs incurred when an abused individual has not received appropriate treatment. Consequently, we have not experienced a great deal of difficulty "making a case" for evaluation and treatment sessions. Another source of funds for treatment is the Victim's Witness program. This program is funded through the state and is available in every state. These funds are to provide medical or psychological treatment (or both) to victims of crime. In order to be eligible for these funds the victim must press charges against the alleged perpetrator. The phone number for Victim's Witness can be found in the white pages of the phone book. The therapist who accepts Victim's Witness funds is required to accept payment at the rate prescribed and provide written reports of treatment goals and progress.

TREATMENT MODALITIES

In cases of intrafamilial abuse, all family members will likely require therapeutic intervention. Usually the child is seen in individual therapy in order to establish a trusting, supportive environment in which to discuss issues. The alleged perpetrator is usually mandated to attend individual therapy in order to explore how she was unable to refrain from aggressing against the child and to come to terms with taking responsibility for her own behaviors. The nonoffending spouse is also frequently recommended to receive therapy in order to explore his feelings about the abuse that took place in the home. Siblings may also receive individual therapy to explore their feelings about the abuse and the effects of the abuse on all the family members.

Child Treatment

The goal of treatment is to help the child counteract practices that lead her not to recognize her own feelings and power. Within the dominant story of abuse, the child is invited to accommodate or "be for others" rather than acknowledge her own needs. As the child feels accepted in the relationship with you, you may begin to explore feelings about others (including the alleged perpetrators), work toward acceptance of all her feelings, and build on her strengths in order to build positive relationships with others.

It is important to note that the child (sometimes despite a history of horrendous abuse) may be very attached, supportive, and protective of his abusive parent. These feelings must also be supported as you work toward separating out the behaviors from the parent. You may sometimes find yourself feeling angry at the parent for the abusive behaviors. Although this is a normal reaction, you must work on separating the behavior from the individual in order to help the child and family do the same. This does not mean denying the parent was "responsible" for the behavior, but quite the opposite.

Building Trust and Safety. Creating a safe environment for the child that allows the child to explore his feelings about the abuse requires that you specify the implicit rules of therapy. The child must know what your limitations are regarding confidentiality and what types of information you will need to share with others. You should discuss the manner in which you receive information about the child (for example, from the child's attorney, social worker, or parent), and the child should be informed about the rules within the therapy room. The room should be a safe place to express feelings, but you may wish to make explicit that throwing objects and hitting are not allowed, as this is behavior that is not respectful of you. Likewise, you should invite the child to let you know if he is not feeling safe. For example, I ask the child to tell me if he does not wish to answer a question I have asked or if he feels uncomfortable at any time.

Exploring Feelings. As mentioned earlier, abused children often do not have a sense of their own feelings, and when asked how they feel they may respond with "Fine" or "I don't know." Sometimes children will respond with a statement of what they have been told by others regarding how they "should" feel. In order for you to help the child rebuild a sense of self, you must be very watchful of your own feelings, so that you do not give the child messages about how to feel. The child may be well practiced in accommodating adults and may be quick to pick up on what an adult wants from her, including how to "feel." You may be tempted to say, "You must be angry," or "You should feel proud of yourself for telling." These well-intentioned statements are made by therapists in an attempt to be supportive, but the effect is that the child is once again informed about what to feel.

You must assess your own intentions and biases. Are you attempting to find more evidence that Father is guilty? Do you feel that Mother did not adequately protect the child? In answering these questions for yourself, you are in a better position to monitor any bias in your language. As the child's therapist, you must focus on the child's need to have room for exploration of her feelings.

One method we like to use is to have the child draw his feelings. In the case that follows, Billy does this to tell more about the feeling of pain he was experiencing. In doing so, he also became aware of other feelings.

BILLY

Billy entered the therapy room for his session, stating, "My knee hurts again." For the last three sessions, Billy had come in with a physical complaint. I asked Billy if he would like to draw his pain. He drew a picture of his leg with a very red knee and referred to the red circle as "pain." I asked him how he felt about "pain" and how "pain" was tripping him up. He described how angry he was at the pain for hurting him and for keeping him from activities. Through his discussion of his feelings toward "pain," Billy was able to explore several other feelings. I would like to note that I did not draw a parallel between these feelings and those he might or might not have had toward his abuser, as I wished to provide an arena for the exploration of feelings, without suggesting how he "may" feel toward someone else. However, several sessions later, Billy said, "Hey, my uncle is like the pain ball. He hurt me, and I am angry at him for hurting me."

Another way we work with children is to help them explore their feelings by having them give us a list of events that occurred that day or over the week and discuss how they felt about the events. As the child becomes more aware of feelings and his right to have his feelings, we may explore how he feels about important events, such as visits with parents (for those children in foster care), or about events in the foster home, and so on. Through this exploration, the child also tends to realize that he may have multiple feelings about events and others and that the behaviors of others do not define them.

Again, art may provide a means of expressing multiple feelings. In the case of Sara, presented next, I asked Sara to draw *all* the feelings she was having. In this way, she was able to experience and recognize that she does have multiple feelings toward others in her life.

SARA

Sara ran to the easel first thing as she entered the therapy room. She wanted to draw how she felt about her foster mother asking her to clean her room prior to coming to the session. She then went on to draw how she felt about an upcoming visit with her mother. She drew her mother with a smile and reported how much she missed her, but drew her face green because of the anger she felt toward her. Sara used different colors to express the multiple feelings she had toward her caregivers. She stated, "This green part is when I am mad at her for hitting, but the blue part is how much I miss her."

Dealing with Guilt, Blame, and Responsibility. As children explore their feelings, they frequently readily identify guilt or self-blame as overriding feelings associated with the abusive experience. For example, one child said, "If I just hadn't slurped my cereal so loud, Dad would not have hit me." Another child stated, "I knew it was wrong, but he promised I could have a car when I turn sixteen." A third child said, "It is my fault for telling, and now my mom had to go to jail." Your goal is to help the child recognize the need for individuals to take responsibility for their own behaviors and to help the child counteract the effects of self-blame and guilt. Easier said than done. In the case that follows, I attempted to help Sammy understand that he was not to blame for his father's drinking but that he was still a powerful individual who is responsible for his own behavior.

SAMMY

Sammy stated in the session, "It is my fault that my dad got drunk and hit me, 'cause I was being too noisy." I asked Sammy if "Noisy" was around all the time, or only sometimes. He stated, "Sometimes at night when Dad comes home, Noisy gets me in trouble." I said that "Noisy" must be extremely powerful to be able to convince someone to drink something. I suggested to Sammy that if he wanted to, we could try an experiment. I placed a glass of water on the table and asked him if he thought "Noisy" could convince me to drink it. Sammy smiled widely. He went over and slammed the door of the room, he yelled, he sang at the top of his voice. Smiling, he said, "I don't think 'Noisy' can make you drink that—only if you pick it up." We discussed that it is his responsibility to keep "Noisy" from getting him a time-out in the foster home but that he is not responsible for what others do.

Fostering Empowerment, Mastery, and Control. Exploring feelings, challenging self-blame, and promoting responsibility for individual behavior all work toward counteracting disempowerment and increasing self-mastery. As therapists, our goal is to help the child regain a sense of self-mastery and to deny the invitation to take on the role of either victim or aggressor. Through the use of puppet or role play, you can explore alternative ways of being powerful. In this play, I ask the child to "direct" me. For example, rather than creating my own role in the play, I ask the child, "What do I say now?" or "What does she do here?" *Please note:* it is important to remember that the use of puppet or role play is a form of "make-believe" and is important to the child's development as a way of enabling him to "try out" ways of being in the world. However, you must guard against having the child recreate abuse scenarios that may or may not have occurred, as this may be confusing to both the child and you.

There are several techniques and play tools (for example, coloring books) available to help children learn about being powerful if they are approached again in an abusive manner. Although adults are more powerful than children, children do have some power. Some of the ways that children can be powerful is to believe that they do not deserve to be harmed. Physically, they can attempt to kick, hit, yell, or run. Many times, however, these options are not open to children. Therefore, we believe it is important to be careful when using empowering techniques that you do not give the message that it is solely up to the child to protect herself. We should encourage children to seek help from others and provide them with resources toward that end with the message that others can and will help.

Increasing Self-Esteem. Many times children will feel negatively about themselves as a result of the abuse and self-blame. You should evaluate their level of depression and risk for self-harm throughout the therapy and intervene accordingly. If the child is in danger of imminent harm, you must put procedures in place to protect the child, including hospitalization if necessary. You should also help the child access the positive feelings she does have about herself and build on these. For example, one child felt good about her ability to do well in school. We explored how she was able to feel good about this accomplishment and how to expand those positive feelings and the recognition of her competencies in other areas of her life.

Working on Socialization. When children have experienced an abusive relationship, they may approach others in ways similar to how they learned to be in that relationship. For example, two brothers who had been physically abused began the session by hitting me with the action figures they had brought with them. Another child, who had been sexually molested, engaged in very seductive behaviors and dress, although only nine years old. These children were also engaging their peers and foster parents in a similar manner.

Needless to say, these behaviors provide a challenge to you as well as to others in the children's lives. One child reported that her peers were rejecting her at school. Another child, who was engaging in seductive behaviors, was rejected by same-age peers but was being approached by the older children in the school.

Teachers feared that she would become a victim of the older children.

You can help children learn alternative ways of connecting with others that may be more age appropriate and respectful. For example, with the child who interacts aggressively, I explain that I am interested in getting to know him but do not want hitting to be part of our relationship. I explain that we can talk and play together but that hitting is not respectful. Again, the use of puppets or role playing is useful in trying out different ways of connecting with others.

It may also be useful to meet with teachers and foster parents to help them understand why these behaviors may exist, to put together behavioral management programs to help the child learn new behaviors, and to encourage the caregivers to resist the invitation to reject these children. These children may bring to any relationship specific qualities of temperament, age, or physical health that may make them difficult to parent and that may have thereby contributed to the abusive relationship. In any case, it is essential that adult caretakers find ways to care for the child in nurturing and safe ways.

Terminating Treatment. This may be an especially difficult time for children, as it may remind them of their many losses. If the child remains in the area, I let him know that I will continue to be available for therapy at a later time if he needs it. Many times, abuse issues may emerge as the child passes through developmental stages, such as adolescence.

When I terminate the therapy with a child, I ask the child how she wants to say goodbye. One child who was moving away and was to continue her therapy with another therapist asked to visit the therapist first so that she could talk over her visit and her feelings with me. She created a list of what she liked to do in therapy to take with her on her visit. This child felt that she had been powerful in our therapy and that she could take her power with her.

Nonoffender Spouse: Individual Therapy

Many times the nonoffending spouse is invited to feel guilty for not "protecting" the child. Sometimes the nonoffending spouse was aware of the abuse and did actually fail to protect the child, due to her own feelings of dependency and inadequacy. Often, however, the spouse was unaware of the abuse and, in some cases, may not believe that the abuse occurred. Again, the therapy should emphasize that adults must take responsibility for their own behavior. If the nonoffending spouse was aware of not protecting the child, this spouse must examine why she felt unable to protect him and what she would need in the future to ensure that she would be able to do so. At the same time, the offender continues to be solely responsible for the offense.

If the spouse was unaware, he is still likely to experience blame from others (from society, the offender, and, perhaps, the victim) as well as self-blame for his inaction. The nonoffending spouse, therefore, is likely to experience symptoms similar to the child: feelings of betrayal, lack of trust, disempowerment, and self-blame.

Offender: Individual Therapy

It should be noted that offenders can restrain themselves and probably have restrained themselves at times from aggressing against others. When we work with these individuals, we seek narrative stories that offer an alternative to the dominant story of abuse. We ask offenders to explore why they do not want to engage in the abusive behaviors, how they have stopped themselves in the past, and what is getting in the way of their self-restraint at present.

This approach is based on the offender's taking responsibility for her behavior and for discontinuing the behavior. These behaviors may frequently provoke you into feeling anger and a desire to "punish" the offender. Again, it is important for you to examine your own feelings and work toward accepting the individual but not "accepting" the abusive behaviors.

Dyadic and Family Therapy

If the child may be reunified with the family or was never removed from the family, dyadic and family therapy are extremely important. The ability to move to dyadic therapy should only occur when the nonoffending spouse is able to support the child, be respectful of the child's perceptions, express empathy for the child, and take responsibility for her own feelings. Some clinicians have warned that this therapy should not occur until the parent is able to "believe" the child. However, we have found it difficult to tell whether, in fact, a parent does believe the child. We prefer to ask the parent if she is able to support the child's perceptions. We have found that sometimes during these dyadic therapies, the child is able to feel safe enough to describe aspects of the abusive behaviors that can help the parent understand (and perhaps, believe) how the child views the alleged abuse.

Nonoffending Spouse and Child Therapy. The therapy with the child and nonoffending spouse should focus on providing a supportive environment to make room for discoveries about each other, build on their competencies, and counteract the effects of secrecy and abuse. Leslie Laing and Amanda Kamsler have written about performing this therapy with mothers and children.

Nonoffending Spouse and Perpetrator. Working through the feelings of betrayal and lack of trust will be extremely important if the parents are to reunite and attempt to bring the family back together. If the offending parent is able to acknowledge his behavior and provide strategies for not allowing abuse to occur in the future, the couple may begin to work on issues that prevent further abuse and provide for positive parenting.

Family Treatment. If the family has moved through the dyadic therapies and reunification appears possible, or if the family was not separated, it is of utmost importance for all family members to be able to discuss the abuse and to have the offender take responsibility for her behavior and be able to assure the family members that abuse will not occur in the future. A brief outline of how the "steps" of this process proceeded with the Brown family is described in the next case example.

THE BROWN FAMILY

I saw Cindy, age six, and Sally, age nine, for approximately six months in "sister" therapy. I also provided conjoint therapy with their foster mother as issues arose in the home. Simultaneously, other professionals were working individually with Mr. Brown (offender) and Ms. Brown (nonoffending spouse), and both parents were seen in group therapy. Mr. Brown had not, at first, acknowledged that he had sexually abused his daughters, but through his individual and group treatment he was able to feel "safe" enough to admit to the abuse.

Because it appeared that the family might be reunited, I began to see the parents as a couple. The therapy went well, and the children were introduced to the family sessions. Mr. Brown was able to admit to his family that he had committed the abusive behaviors. He also demonstrated that he had developed coping strategies and established environmental safeguards which would ensure that he would never hurt them again. This family was reunited and followed for several years, with no evidence of recidivism.

Although the Brown family was able to be reunited successfully, this is not always the outcome. Many times the family is not able to be reunited. Sometimes families are reunited and the children are abused again. The treating professionals and Child

Protective Services workers are in the unenviable position of attempting to provide information to the court to help the judge make decisions that are in the best interest of the child. CPS is mandated to work toward family preservation and is motivated to provide services so that families can potentially be reunited. However, methods and research regarding the evaluation of a family's readiness for reunification, the prediction of the family's potential for dangerousness, and the outcomes of treatment are far from adequate.

TREATMENT OUTCOME

Outcome research is inconclusive with regard to treatment effectiveness but indicates that therapy appears to be helpful, especially during the acute adjustment period for children who are most at risk. Kim Oates and Donald Bross conducted a literature review of the last decade of treatment outcome studies of physically abused children. Only twenty-five papers met their criteria of having more than five subjects, pre- and post-testing, and a comparison group for treatment. The programs reviewed indicated that therapeutic day care was useful in promoting developmental skills. However, most studies had very little or no follow-up, so it was difficult to determine if treatment gains were sustained. Research in this area is hampered by funding problems for treatment and research programs and by the difficulty in following families over time.

Treatment outcome data on offenders also indicate mixed success. The percentage of recidivism or reabuse following treatment has ranged from 10 percent to 30 percent in some samples. Some studies have found evidence that family factors and severity of maltreatment may mediate treatment effects. Parents who remained in treatment longer (and thus may have been more compliant) appeared to show the most positive treatment outcome. Again, lack of long-term follow-up data makes it difficult to know if treatment effects are sustained.

MUNCHAUSEN BY PROXY

TOMMY

The nurse turns to me and groans, "Tommy is back, and his diarrhea is worse than ever. I wish we could find out what is wrong with this poor child." His mother, wide-eyed, is at the nursing station stating that they came to the emergency room this morning when Tommy woke up with severe diarrhea once again. She is close to tears, and she reports that she is at her wit's end. Tommy has missed so much school due to his chronic diarrhea that he has a home tutor. Later that day, the lab results indicate strong evidence of laxative in Tommy's stool. Tommy's mother is not allowed to visit him without a nurse present. His diarrhea resolves for the first time in many years. He is able to return to school full-time.

Munchausen by proxy (MBP) describes a form of child abuse in which someone (usually the mother) persistently fabricates or creates symptoms on behalf of another person (usually her child), causing that person to be regarded as medically ill or psychiatrically disturbed. The parent tends to relate a fictitious history and may also induce signs and symptoms of illness, thus subjecting the child to extensive hospitalizations, invasive treatments, and painful procedures. This leads to suffering by the child and sometimes permanent disablement, and may evolve into actually causing illness and death. As I (Sanders) have written about more extensively elsewhere, when the child is older she may be invited to "collude" or participate in the illness story.

As in other forms of abuse, the psychological effect on the child is that the child is objectified and sometimes treated as an "illness" rather than as an individual. In this form of abuse, however, the child may be unaware of the abusive behavior on the part of her parent. From the child's perspective, the parent may appear very caring and supportive.

Most of what we know about this form of child abuse has been obtained through single-case research. As for other forms of abuse, research evidence indicates that following the removal of the child and the treatment period, some parents have reabused the child (or another child in the family). There is also some limited evidence that treatment has apparently been successful in some cases, with no reoccurrence of the MBP behaviors after one to four years.

The determination that MBP behaviors may have occurred is made by the medical team in consultation with psychiatrists and psychologists. Following the identification of MBP behaviors, the treatment team must make some decisions as to how to maintain the safety of the child. The team may decide that separating the parent and child is necessary in order to determine whether the ill child is able to return to health once she is out of the parent's care.

Whether reunification occurs or not, it is recommended that the parents be required to engage in a medical monitoring plan. This plan is designed to quickly identify any reoccurrence of MBP behaviors that may take place with present or future children. Parents *must* agree to authorize all medical treatment through a primary physician (preferably the physician who identified the MBP behaviors) with a second physician acting as back-up, such that *all* treatment is authorized by these two physicians only. In essence, the physician team agrees to take on the responsibility of monitoring the family's access to medical care throughout the childhood years of all the present and future children.

Our treatment approach with individuals who have allegedly engaged in MBP behaviors is similar to the approach already described in treating individuals who have abused their children in other ways. We elicit the narrative of how the parent was invited into the MBP behaviors, we encourage the parent to take responsibility for her behavior, and we develop the alternative story in which the MBP behaviors do not occur. Through the construction of these stories, we attempt to help the parent take responsibility for her actions and develop coping strategies and safeguards that will prevent the abuse from occurring in the future.

As previously described, the offending parent may engage in couples therapy and in dyadic therapies with the children as the family moves toward reunification. If reunification is not possible, the child would not be included in the dyadic therapy with the offender.

The incidence of reported abuse is extremely high, and the needs of individuals who have experienced abuse, as well as those who have perpetrated abuse, are immense. Psychological therapy is often indicated for all members of the family in which the abuse occurred. Our treatment approach is built on a model of etiology that appreciates the complexity of contributing factors and guides a thorough assessment of those factors prior to treatment. The therapy method we use is a narrative approach which emphasizes that the offending adult understands his behavior and takes responsibility for it while at the same time seeing it within the context of complex interactions. In addition, we work to develop an understanding of the circumstances in which the offender does not abuse, in order to help him develop an alternative story of himself and how he can cope and behave in benevolent ways. This therapeutic approach offers a means of avoiding the quagmires of self-blame and reproach while enhancing self-understanding and responsibility and developing respectful and nurturing ways of behaving.

The child treatment focuses on counteracting the negative effects of abuse, co-constructing a self-story of health, and rebuilding relationships in which abusive behaviors do not occur. Prospective studies have found that being a victim of abuse places the child at more risk for engaging in criminal and violent behavior in his adult life. This finding underlines the need to provide appropriate treatment and support to abused children and their families as an attempt to break this cycle of violence.

NOTES

P. 189, *The National Center on Child Abuse and Neglect:* National Center on Child Abuse and Neglect. (1994). *State statues related to child abuse and neglect: 1994.* Washington, DC: U.S. Department of Health and Human Services.

P. 190, *In 1962, Kempe, Silverman, Steele, Droegemueller, and Silver:* Kempe, C. H., Silverman, F. N., Steele, B. F., Droegemueller, W., & Silver, H. (1962). The battered child syndrome. *Journal of the American Medical Association, 181,* 17–24.

P. 190, *battered-child syndrome was affirmed in the legal arena:* People v. Jackson, 18 Cal. App. 3d 504, 95 Cal. Rptr. 919 (1971).

P. 190, *Child Abuse Prevention and Treatment Act:* Myers, J. E. B. (1992). *Legal issues in child abuse and neglect.* Thousand Oaks, CA: Sage.

P. 190, *The definitions of reportable child abuse . . . in each state's penal code:* Cal. Penal Code Section 11165.1(c) (West 1993).

P. 191, *The law requires that mandated reporters immediately call CPS:* Myers, J. E. B. (1992). *ibid.*

P. 191, *model developed by Jay Belsky:* Belsky, J. (1993). Etiology of child maltreatment: A developmental-ecological analysis. *Psychological Bulletin, 114*(3), 413–434.

P. 192, *"There is no one pathway to these disturbances in parenting":* Belsky, J. (1993). *ibid.*

P. 192, *Michael White's narrative model of psychotherapy:* White, M., & Epston, D. (1990). *Narrative means to therapeutic ends.* New York: Norton.

P. 193, *the possible effects of abuse on the developing child:* Becker, J. V., Alpert, J. L., BigFoot, D. S., Bonner, B. L., Geddie, L. F., Henggeler, S. W., Kaufman, K. L., & Walker, C. E. (1995). Empirical research on child abuse treatment: Report by the child abuse and neglect treatment working group, American Psychological Association. *Journal of Clinical Child Psychology, 24*(Suppl.), 23–46.

P. 194, *school difficulties:* Salinger, S., Kaplan, S., Pelcovitz, D., Samit, C., & Kreiger, R. (1984). Parent and teacher assessment of children's behavior in child maltreating families. *Journal of the American Academy of Child Psychiatry, 23,* 458–464.

P. 194, *delinquent or violent . . . depressed and suicidal:* Widom, C. S. (1989). Does violence beget violence? A critical examination of the literature. *Psychological Bulletin, 106*(1), 3–28.

P. 194, *sexually and physically abused children may commonly experience . . . (PTSD) symptoms:* Briere, J. N. (1992). *Child abuse trauma.* Thousand Oaks, CA: Sage.

P. 194, *Maxfield and Widom:* Maxfield, M. G., & Widom, C. S. (1996). The cycle of violence: Revisited six years later. *Archives of Pediatrics and Adolescent Medicine, 150*(4), 390–395.

P. 194, *Some of the factors associated with increased distress:* Nash, M. R., Zivney, O. A., & Hulsey, T. (1993). Characteristics of sexual abuse associated with greater psychological impairment among children. *Child Abuse and Neglect, 17,* 401–408.

P. 195, *Mennen found:* Mennen, F. E. (1993). Evaluation of risk factors in childhood sexual abuse. *Journal of American Academy of Child and Adolescent Psychiatry, 32*(5), 934–939.

P. 195, *Coffey found:* Coffey, P., Leitenberg, H., Henning, K., Turner, T., & Bennett, R. T. (1996). Mediators of the long-term impact of child sexual abuse: Perceived stigma, betrayal, powerlessness, and self-blame. *Child Abuse and Neglect, 20*(5), 447–455.

P. 195, *family and sociocultural factors . . . or neglectful events:* Herrenkohl, E. C., Herrenkohl, R. C., Rupert, L. J., Egolf, B. P., & Lutz, J. G. (1995). Risk factors for behavioral dysfunction: The relative impact of maltreatment, SES, physical health problems, cognitive ability, and quality of parent-child interaction. *Child Abuse and Neglect, 19,* 191–203.

P. 206, *Leslie Laing and Amanda Kamsler have written:* Laing, L., & Kamsler, A. (1992). Putting an end to secrecy: Therapy with mothers and children following disclosure of child sexual abuse. In Durrant, M., & White, C. (Eds.), *Ideas for therapy with sexual abuse.* South Australia: Dulwich Centre Publications.

P. 208, *Kim Oates and Donald Bross:* Oates, R. K., & Bross, D. C. (1995). What have we learned about treating child physical abuse: A literature review of the last decade. *Child Abuse and Neglect, 19*(4), 463–473.

P. 208, *recidivism . . . ranged from 10 to 30 percent:* Lutzker, J. R., & Rice, J. M. (1984). Project 12-ways: Measuring outcome of a large in-home service for treatment and prevention of child abuse and neglect. *Child Abuse and Neglect, 8,* 519–524; Rivara, F. P. (1985). Physical abuse in children under two: A study of therapeutic outcomes. *Child Abuse and Neglect, 9,* 81–87.

P. 208, *family factors . . . may mediate treatment effects:* Pelcovitz, D., Kaplan, S., Samit, C., Krieger, R., & Cornelius, D. (1984). Adolescent abuse: Family structure and implications for treatment. *Journal of the American Academy of Child and Adolescent Psychiatry, 32,* 85–90.

P. 208, *Parents who remained in treatment longer:* Land, H. M. (1986). Child abuse: Differential diagnosis, differential treatment. *Child Welfare, 65,* 33–44.

P. 209, *she may be invited to "collude"* . . . *the illness story:* Sanders, M. J. (1995). Symptom coaching: Factitious disorder by proxy with older children. *Clinical Psychology Review, 15*(5), 423–442.

P. 210, *treatment has apparently been successful in some cases:* Sanders, M. J. (1996). Narrative family treatment of Munchausen by proxy: A successful case. *Families, Systems, & Health, 14*(3), 315–329.

8

EATING DISORDERS

Tamara M. Altman and James Lock

MARY

Mary, nine, was referred to us for evaluation by her pediatrician for weight loss and "picky" eating, for which no medical cause could be found. She arrived at our clinic with her mother and older brother. She was very thin and pale, and was dressed in a short dress and white stockings. Her appearance was exceptionally neat, and her thin blond hair was pulled back tightly in a small, perfectly shaped bun. She spoke very little during the interview, and when she did, she was barely audible. Her answers were short, and her voice carried little emotion.

Mary's mother reported that Mary had always been a demanding child. As an infant, she had trouble sleeping through the night and kept her mother awake nursing her until Mary was over a year old. Mary's mother had decided that she would no longer breast-feed Mary after she was six months old, but switching to formula did not help Mary sleep through the night any better. As a toddler, Mary continued to demand much of her mother's time and energy, and when she didn't receive it, she threw loud tantrums. At this point Mary was a "chubby" child, and her mother began "helping" Mary eat better.

During her early childhood, Mary became moody and irritable. She was anxious, and she cried bitterly whenever her mother left her at the day-care center. When she reunited with her mother, she was angry and sullen, often ignoring her. Mary had little interest in her father, and he seemed preoccupied with her older brother. Mary remained "chubby" as a toddler, and the family encouraged her to be more athletic "like your brother." Mary's mother started doing exercises with Mary, which was something that Mary enjoyed.

By the time Mary started kindergarten, she had learned to control her temper and "neediness" but had become increasingly competitive with peers. Although during the early elementary school years she received good marks and was viewed positively by her teachers, she developed few friendships and spent most of her free time doing homework. Toward the end of third grade, Mary stopped eating desserts, and Mary's mother praised her for this because she felt Mary was overweight. Mary began to demand salads, and her mother noticed that when Mary took her lunch to school, she returned with it only half eaten. Eventually, Mary stopped eating with the family except under great pressure to do so.

Over the following six months, Mary ate less and began to exercise vigorously. Her mother confronted her about her behaviors, and they began to have screaming fights. Her mother demanded that she eat in front of her and weighed Mary daily. Still, Mary continued to lose weight. Mary's pediatrician referred her for evaluation at our clinic. Mary's mother resisted this idea and delayed bringing Mary to the clinic for several months after the initial referral.

As child psychiatrists and researchers who work in an academic setting that has a long history of treating children and adults with eating disorders, we are naturally referred many patients of all ages with eating problems of all types. Our perspective is one that we have developed in the context of both clinical and research activities. Because we have been in the business of taking care of children with eating disorders at Stanford for a long time, we have the benefit of a lot of collected institutional wisdom that we also use routinely in our treatment. Our perspective on working with school-age children with eating disorders is one that is fundamentally based on a developmental understanding of childhood. This means that our treatment incorporates the intellectual, emotional, and psychological capacities that are generally in place for school-age children, and includes an appreciation of the importance of family, peers, and group standards during the school-age years. Every treatment that we suggest in this chapter is described in terms that are specific to the school-age child and takes into account the developmental issues that are key for school-age children.

Mary's story is a typical example of a school-age child with symptoms of an eating disorder. Today, eating disorders are becoming recognized as a major health problem among young people. Although it is more common for eating problems to surface during adolescence, we also work with school-age children with eating disorders (and those who display risk factors for eating disorders). Although it is quite rare to see school-age children with full-blown eating disorders (Anorexia Nervosa occurs less than 10 percent of the time in children under the age of eleven, and other eating problems, such as fear of swallowing, occur in less than 1 percent of school-age children), subclinical concerns regarding weight and dieting occur in close to 50 percent of school-age girls. Working with the children in our clinic has provided us with a better understanding of the issues that young people deal with and of the link between these types of issues and eating problems.

In this chapter, we take a look at the prevalence of symptoms and risk factors associated with eating disorders in school-age children. We provide an overview on the prevalence, diagnosis, assessment, and treatment of eating disorders in school-age children and discuss the opportunity for preventive efforts that exists with this age group.

DO EATING DISORDERS APPEAR THIS EARLY?

For many of the school-age children we work with, weight concerns and weight control behaviors are a large part of their lives. Researchers have been telling us for some time now that these issues are important for young people. One study found that 45 percent of third through sixth graders indicated a desire to be thinner, and 37 percent of the children reported having tried to lose weight. More recent findings show a link between fourth- and fifth-grade girls' weight concerns and the importance that their peers put on weight and eating, on how much they try to look like girls and women on television or in magazines, and on their body mass index (weight-height). Although there is a clear gender difference with regard to weight concerns, dieting, and eating disorders among adolescents and adults (girls outnumber boys approximately ten to one with regard to developing eating disorders), such concerns and behaviors are more equally distributed among school-age boys and girls. We have seen both boys and girls with eating problems. We also know that even more prevalent among this age group are the risk factors that play a role in the development of eating disorders.

RISK FACTORS FOR EATING DISORDERS

Risk factors for eating disorders include biological, psychological and behavioral, familial, sociocultural, and peer domains.

Biological Factors

There are certain biological factors that we do not have much control over—being male or female and or of a particular body shape—that are associated with eating disorders. This shouldn't be surprising, as these kind of factors very clearly influence how we think of ourselves and our bodies. Other biological factors that are not considered here, such as genetic vulnerabilities and metabolic abnormalities, may also play important roles in the development and maintenance of eating disorders.

Gender. Eating disorders and the risk factors associated with them are more common in girls than boys. More than 90 percent of anorectics and 80 percent of bulimics are female. For girls, the importance of looking good and staying thin tends to be higher than for boys. When asked about the positive things about being a girl, one school-age girl that we talked with could only reply, "You can be pretty. And you can, well, that's all."

Body Weight and Height. School-age girls who are heavier than average for their age are more likely to feel bad about their bodies and to want to lose weight. These girls are also more at risk for eating disorders. Many girls from a community sample told us that girls who are heavier are more likely to be teased about their weight, feel bad about themselves, and be on weight-loss diets.

Puberty. Puberty (especially early onset of puberty) may be a risk factor for the development of eating disorders. Puberty brings about physical and emotional changes that are often confusing and a bit frightening. As one young girl put it, "It's sort of scary because you don't know what's happening to you, and it's like there's something wrong with you."

Psychological and Behavioral Factors

We have seen many psychological and behavioral factors associated with eating disorders. Patterns that school-age children begin to develop in terms of how they think about themselves, how they think about what happens to them, and how they behave in everyday life and in response to specific situations set the course for the pathways of their lives. For example, children who are already concerned with their weight and who feel they need to be perfect in everything they do are more likely to develop eating disorders.

Early Feeding Behaviors. We have found that children's feeding difficulties at very young ages are associated with later eating problems. A number of the school-age eating disorder patients we see have experienced some type of feeding difficulty since birth. One example is a ten-year-old boy we treated in our clinic. He began to vomit, at the age of three, during times when he was anxious. He developed a pattern of vomiting under stressful situations that proved increasingly embarrassing and dysfunctional as he entered school.

More commonly, children and parents develop early struggles around food intake. This often occurs during the toddler years. Parents feed their children to "help them grow" but end up with children who do not understand when they are hungry or not hungry. This can lead to problems with weight and food in the school-age years and beyond.

Weight Concerns. Some individuals experience such excessive weight concerns that they feel driven to use drastic measures to lose weight. Excessive weight concern predicts the onset of eating disorders in adolescent girls. One fifth-grade girl we talked with listed "weight and how we look" as the biggest problems for girls. An eleven-year-old girl we saw in our clinic described how, when she was only six years old, she used to compare her thighs with other girls' thighs.

Dieting. Many times we have seen that what may begin as a harmless cutting back on a few calories or avoiding certain foods can turn into very restrictive behaviors that can lead to bingeing and purging. By age thirteen, 80 percent of girls have already been on a weight-loss diet. In response to the question "What do you think are the most important issues for girls your age?" a fourth-grade girl from a local school said, "Looking good for boys and, if you're overweight, watching what you eat." It's not just girls, though. One nine-year-old boy who had severe asthma requiring treatment with prednisone (which can cause weight gain) became so anxious about his weight that he began restricting all fats and sugars from his diet.

Personality Traits. Those of us who work with anorexic individuals know that they can often be compliant, perfectionistic, goal oriented, shy, and sometimes obsessive. On the other hand, we know that bulimic individuals tend to be impulsive and less concerned with the impressions they convey to others. Such personality traits are established during the school-age years. A typical example of a school-age child with a restrictive or anorexic style is Suzy, who in addition to "perfecting" her weight was also a champion swimmer, straight-A student, ballet dancer, and compliant child.

Depression. Our clinical and research experiences suggest that children who are depressed are more likely to develop eating disorders. Also, family studies and our clinical experience show a high incidence of affective disorders among family members of patients with eating disorders. The nine-year-old asthmatic boy we mentioned earlier also suffered from a depression. He was chronically worried about his asthma and felt hopeless about ever getting over it. He often complained that life was not worth living. When he started restricting calories to lose weight, he began to have a feeling of control that, although illusory, temporarily disguised his depressed feelings.

Stress and Coping. Children who have been exposed to a greater number of stressful life events than is normal for their age are also at risk for developing eating disorders. Similarly, individuals who are not equipped to deal successfully with challenges in their lives may also be at risk. Eating-disordered behaviors can seem to provide a controllable, safe escape from other stressors.

We see many patients in our clinic who have suffered through traumatic events, and their eating problems are often related to their struggles with these experiences. Sexual and physical abuse are two such experiences. School-age children who have endured sexual or physical abuse and have not successfully worked through their trauma may develop eating-disordered behaviors in an attempt to exert control over their bodies. One example of this was an eight-year-old girl who could not swallow. She said she felt she would suffocate if she tried to drink or eat anything.

It turned out that this little girl had been forced to orally copulate with her mother's boyfriend over a period of several months when she was four years old.

Family Factors

School-age children rely on their families for support, guidance, and nurturing. When there are problems related to the family environment, there may be negative effects on children's social, intellectual, and physical development. The level of family disturbance is often high among children with eating disorders, and most of the patients we see in our clinic have some type of family problem that must be addressed during treatment.

Family Dysfunction. The family dynamics of our anorectic patients are often characterized by a failure to individuate from an enmeshed and overprotective family. The bulimic individuals we have seen tend to describe their families as providing insufficient encouragement for independence, low tolerance for the open expression of emotions, and high levels of chaos and conflict. The family of one ten-year-old girl who developed bulimia is an example of this. This third-generation Asian-American family consisted of five girls—ages four to ten—and two parents. No regular meals were served in the family. Food was sometimes not in the house. Mother and father did not speak to each other, though the mother was furious at her husband for leaving the family for long hours at work. The combination of a lack of nurturance, both physical and emotional, with an inability to express conflict set the stage for bulimia to develop in the oldest daughter.

Parental Preoccupation with Weight and Eating. Parental attitudes toward weight and eating influence children's attitudes. When a parent is preoccupied with his or her own thinness and food intake, the child is at increased risk for the development of eating disorders. Imitation of parental weight preoccupations and eating habits seem to be one way in which a young person can gain desired attention and respect from a parent. One girl related her experiences of dieting with her mom: "Every night I go jogging with my mom. . . . We stay healthy, we eat salads every night, and we eat vegetables."

Attachment and Separation Issues. Insecure attachment styles are characterized by interpersonal difficulties, which are often recognized in eating-disordered individuals. School-age children with eating problems and weight concerns are more likely to feel insecure about their relationships than are individuals without eating problems and with fewer weight concerns. The following case illustrates the importance of attachment and separation issues in school-age-onset eating disorders.

SALLY

Sally was born with severe scoliosis, and at the age of nine she was scheduled to have major surgery. She began to eat less and started vomiting. She denied any attempt to lose weight, but she quickly became very malnourished. In addition to these problems, Sally's sister had been sexually abused by Sally's father, and Sally's mother had been sexually abused by her own father. Sally was aware of these problems but had not been abused herself. In reaction to these problems, Sally's mother had at times been very close to Sally, but at other times she had left Sally in others' care for months at a time.

On review of this case, it was clear that Sally was depressed and anxious about separation from her mother. Her own dependency needs were managed inadequately by her mother. Sally anticipated pain, disability, and perhaps even paralysis in conjunction with the surgery. Taken together, problems with attachment, dependency, and anticipated surgical trauma expressed themselves by Sally's developing an eating disorder. Unlike what is often the case for older girls, she did not experience body image problems; she was not trying to undo or prevent the onset of adolescence nor was she in a struggle with her mother over developmental adolescent problems. Instead, she developed an eating disorder partly because of poor parenting and attachment relationships in the context of the severe stressor of a traumatic surgery.

Family History of Eating Problems. Having a family member with a history of an eating disorder places individuals at risk for eating disorders. Genetic and modeling issues may help explain this association.

Sociocultural Factors

"There's this one model I like [on the television show *Beverly Hills 90210*]. . . . I want to be her when I grow up. . . . She's really pretty, and I like her hair" (Jessica, nine years old). From television sitcoms to magazines in the supermarket, we are constantly receiving images telling us that to be thin and beautiful is to be happy and successful. Such images tell children that their appearance should be a main priority and that they should focus on having a very thin body.

Peer Factors

What a child's friends are doing and thinking about their weight and eating can be very influential. School-age girls will change their eating habits in order to appear in a more positive light with their peers. As one girl explains, when a girl is around boys she "probably eats less than she normally eats, because she probably wouldn't want them to make fun of her." This brings up the issue of teasing. Teasing about weight and shape occurs frequently in the school-age years and is probably associated with children's developing unhealthy weight regulation behaviors. When we asked a fourth-grade girl from our community sample what it means when a boy calls a girl fat, she responded, "[It means] that you're ugly and fat and no one wants to be around you." As we can see, teasing can be hurtful and is often linked with feelings of low self-esteem and body image problems. Girls sometimes try to lose weight when their bodies are the source of teasing, and they may see behaviors (even eating-disordered behaviors) that can possibly eliminate such teasing as advantageous.

How Risk Factors Work

In our experience, we have seen that risk factors tend to have a cumulative effect. Each new factor that gets added to a child's life poses greater stress and makes it more likely that pathology will express itself. In many of the cases we have seen, a precipitating event—one that pushes the child beyond what she can handle—transforms the risk that has accumulated over the years into an eating disorder. The risk factors our patients have experienced play varying roles during the different developmental phases of their lives, from childhood through adulthood. For example, family factors are more significant in the school-age years, and sociocultural ideals regarding thinness and beauty are more salient in the adolescent years.

DIAGNOSES AND ASSESSMENT

The *DSM-IV* lists the following criteria for Anorexia Nervosa: being underweight, having an intense fear of gaining weight or becoming fat, experiencing body image disturbances, and, in postmenarcheal females, experiencing the absence of at least three consecutive menstrual cycles. Bulimia Nervosa is marked by bingeing (intake of a large amount of food in a short period of time and a feeling of lack of control over eating); purging (self-induced vomiting; misuse of laxatives, diuretics, or enemas; fasting; or intense exercise); and placing excessive importance on body weight and shape.

An individual who has some, but not all, of the symptoms just listed may be diagnosed with Eating Disorder Not Otherwise Specified (EDNOS). Because school-age children with eating disturbances are often at the early stages of a disorder, and many of the criteria for Anorexia Nervosa and Bulimia Nervosa are most appropriate for postpubertal individuals, we find that the EDNOS category is of great importance when considering younger people, and we often use it with our school-age patients.

Because the *DSM-IV* was not developed for school-age children, we urge you to be cautious if you use this assessment tool with children. There are differences between school-age children with eating disorders and older individuals with eating disorders. For example, some young children we have treated have abstained from liquid intake as well as from food intake. Another major problem that we have come across is the identification of whether or not a child is underweight. A weight loss of 25 percent of body weight is the typical criteria for adolescents and adults. Because school-age children have proportionally less total body fat before weight loss than do adolescents and adults, a lower percentage of weight loss for children will produce detrimental health effects.

There is some debate about whether eating disorders should be assessed in a continuous or categorical fashion. In terms of school-age children, we think that a more continuous diagnostic system may be especially useful, as the symptoms that this age group exhibits may be less severe forms of adolescents' and adults' symptoms.

The overall elements of assessment for any psychiatric disorder are included in our assessments of school-age children being evaluated for eating disorders. These elements include a parent interview, an interview and mental status exam of the child, and a family interview. These interviews may require more than one session, depending on the amount of information to collect and the obstacles to collecting it. We also seek information from pediatricians, teachers, and other significant family members.

Parent Interview

Assessment usually begins by meeting with the parents. We have found that meeting with the parents first often provides us with a context for the child's behaviors.

When taking a history from the parents of a child with a suspected eating disorder, begin by taking a complete feeding history. We think it is best to start from birth and ask questions about how the child did with nursing, whether he was breast fed or bottle fed, how and when solid foods were introduced, and how solid foods were tolerated. In addition, ask about the emotional context of these early feedings. One mother of a nine-year-old described the early period of nursing her daughter as "hell for me. She woke up at all hours, then bit me and ended the whole thing by spitting up all over me." For this mother-daughter pair, the relationship around food never improved. It is also important to ask about the child's birth weight and his weight gain process during infancy. Often there are parental concerns about chubbiness even from the child's earliest infancy.

Next, proceed to questions about feeding and weight issues in the toddler period. We have found that many parents of children who later develop eating disorders describe battles of control over food during these early years. The mother, whose eight-year-old boy vomited frequently, described their feeding sessions as a "battleground." She described leaving him in his highchair for an hour after meals to get him to eat. This usually failed, so she often resorted to coaxing him to eat anything—usually sweet cereal—so that he would "have something in him."

Continue to seek information about eating and weight concerns in early childhood and the years when the child started school. We have noticed that this is a time when the child's problems may "go underground" and are less evident to the parents. At times, parents do admit to their having a more concentrated concern with the child's weight. Such concern is often a reaction to the prospect that their child will be teased at school if she is overweight. Often the parents may directly or indirectly support the development of weight concerns by rewarding the child for not eating or for exercising. The mother of a nine-year-old boy who started exercising and limiting calories had bought him a Stairmaster out of her concern that he would be teased if he gained weight. She felt it would be good for him if he stayed thin.

The most recent history of eating patterns is also important to obtain. Has the child cut out fats? Sugar? Meat? Protein? Has she cut out particular foods, or is she indiscriminate in her behaviors? How long have the behaviors been going on, and how much weight has been lost? Does the child eat in front of the family? Are there special food rituals (bowls or special utensils)? Does the child hoard food in special hiding places? You should also ask questions about vomiting, exercise, and binge eating. These questions help you gauge the degree of current difficulty and the need for acute intervention.

You should also ask parents about symptoms of depression and anxiety disorders in their child, as eating behaviors may be a manifestation of these disturbances. If such symptoms are present, we urge you to explore the relationship between the eating behaviors and these other disorders, because this relationship is likely to be crucial to your making the correct diagnosis and treatment.

The parent interview can be completed by taking a history from the parents on their own eating behaviors and weight histories. Sometimes these interviews should be conducted with each parent individually because many parents have not disclosed relevant eating and weight experiences to their partners. It has not been at all unusual for us to find that food and weight issues have been and currently are major issues for one or both of the parents. When this is the case, it is important that it be recognized as a probable complication of treatment.

Child Interview

Although, in general, school-age children can often tell you a lot, by the time a child is referred to you, he probably has learned what not to say and may mislead you about his eating behaviors and weight concerns. One particularly bright child, the son of a physician, described his weight loss as a "matter of health." He said he knew that fat and sugar were bad for him, and he simply had stopped eating them. This might have been more believable if he hadn't also restricted complex carbohydrates and fluids as well. Still, with a cooperative child you can expect her to answer questions about what she eats, how much she eats, when she eats, what she doesn't eat, and her thoughts about weight. She may also tell you about how she thinks she compares to others and why it is important to her to be thin. In our experience, most school-age children have not been able to give much information on the larger family context of their problems.

In this interview, it is important to ask questions about other psychiatric symptoms, such as depression, anxiety, or problems resulting from being apart from either parent, and whether there is any relationship between these problems and the child's current eating behaviors. Questions about sexual and physical abuse should also be part of this interview.

Our mental status examinations with school-age children with eating disorders often reveal preoccupations with food and weight and sometimes distorted body perceptions. The presence of other problems—with concentration, depressed affect, or psychotic thinking—increases the possibility of the child's having another disorder.

Family Interview

Family interviews are sometimes difficult to arrange, and setting them up can in itself be instructive. When families avoid the interview, or schedule and then don't show up, or when all members do not attend, you learn a lot about the family's functioning. Any of these behaviors increases the likelihood that problems in the family as a whole are contributing to the disordered eating behaviors.

The focus of our family interviews for assessment is to ascertain the basic dynamics of the family unit: Who sides with whom? Who works well with whom? In addition to these basic elements, we want to find out, if possible, what the role of the eating disorder is in the family. Does it take the focus away from other problems? Does anyone benefit from the eating disorder?

Does it keep the family together? But getting answers to these questions can be stressful. The conflicts in these families are usually deep and long standing. When these conflicts are revealed, try to remain gentle and caring. This can be difficult for you if a family is angling to get you to take sides or to ignore the proverbial elephant in the room.

Pediatrician

In cases of suspected eating disorders, it is important to have contact with the child's pediatrician, because he or she often has a more objective history of weight and feeding problems. Unfortunately, many pediatricians with whom we work have very little knowledge about eating disorders and require assistance in knowing what will help you in doing an assessment. Most of them can readily provide you with a height and weight chart and history. What they usually cannot tell you is how the patient was weighed (dressed or undressed, with or without shoes or other unknown weighty objects). Often they can tell you if there is evidence of chronic vomiting, because of potassium levels and throat irritation, but they are less likely to know if the child has been concerned about his weight. A pediatrician called to refer a patient to us one day and said, "I don't know what to do about this girl—I tell her to eat, and she just won't do it. She doesn't seem to be mentally retarded, but I can't get through to her."

The time you spend talking to the child's pediatrician will pay off, as he or she is likely to be a critical player in the ultimate treatment plan. The most important part of the interview with the pediatrician is to learn of any medical problems that may be contributing to weight loss and the child's current medical stability.

Teachers and Others

It has been our experience in working with school-age children that they often behave very differently within their families than they do with peers or with other adults. In order to assess a child's skills and behaviors, it is important to discuss both his academic and social performance at school.

In general, the restrictive, anorectic patient usually excels in academics and other areas related to individual performance, but does poorly with social skills; on the other hand, those with other kinds of eating disorders tend to do less well academically but may be more popular with peers. It is often more important to obtain information about the child's interpersonal skills than about his academic performance. It can be difficult for teachers to appreciate or believe that one of their prized students has emotional problems. One teacher we spoke to about an eight-year-old girl with a restrictive eating pattern became so enraged at the idea that this "bright and talented" child needed emotional help, she hung up the phone in disgust. It took some doing to get her to understand how serious the problem might become.

PSYCHOLOGICAL AND MEDICAL TREATMENTS

Having completed your interviews and collected information from pediatricians and teachers, you can now develop a formulation and a treatment plan. Treatment of a school-age child with an eating disorder usually involves both psychological and medical treatments. Psychological treatment includes the first contact, family therapy, individual therapy, and behavioral intervention. Medical treatment includes nutritional education and medical monitoring. In this next section, we discuss each of these modalities and give examples of how to work in each. We also discuss issues of countertransference and problems with managed care.

Psychological Treatment

Working therapeutically with school-age children requires an appreciation of the basic psychodynamics of this developmental period. Freud called this period "latency" because it appeared to him that the strong sexual and aggressive impulses characteristic of younger children went underground during these years. It is perhaps better to understand this period as one in which sexual and aggressive impulses are not inactive but rather are managed differently and more indirectly.

A child who is successful during this period of life needs to establish ways to manage sexual and aggressive impulses that, although still present, cannot be directly expressed because the child is not sexually mature or physically large enough to take on adult behaviors. The child who displays eating-disordered behaviors is likely to experience difficulty in achieving this ability. Therefore, your aim is to assist the child in developing these capacities. The following case example serves to illustrate the various components of psychological treatment.

MARK

Mark was an eight-year-old boy referred to us for evaluation of an atypical eating disorder. He refused to eat any vegetables or meat, and his diet had consisted almost exclusively of cheese and cereals for more than two years.

First Contact

Mark was thin and pale, but he had no acute medical problems. Mark's parents reported that he had problems with nightmares, tantrums, oppositional behaviors, sadness, and suicidal ideation. Mark was the middle child of an intact family with professional parents, a twelve-year-old brother, and a two-year-old sister.

Although it was apparent that Mark suffered from a depression in addition to his eating disorder, the symptoms of the eating disorder antedated the depression and represented, to a certain extent, a separate set of problems from the depression. Still, the more immediate concern was Mark's depression, and treatment began by providing an opportunity to use play therapy to express Mark's conflicts with his older brother, younger sister, and parents.

Treatment for depression in this age group is described in Chapter Three, but suffice it to say here, Mark responded to this increased support, and his depressive symptoms and irritability improved greatly. Nonetheless, his eating patterns remained atypical. To help him, we developed a three-pronged approach that included simultaneous family therapy, individual play therapy, and behavioral therapy.

FAMILY THERAPY

Mark and his family (except his younger sister) arrived on time, though harried, for our first family session. Mark's mother had called us several times with anxiety about the family therapy because of problems between her and her husband. Within the first few minutes of the family session, several major problems became evident. The first was that the family was overwhelmed with the needs of all of its members. No one felt well taken care of, with the possible exception of Mark's father. The older son reported feeling neglected since Mark had started therapy. Mark's mother appeared depressed and anxious. The second problem was that the family used chaos and the overwhelming number of "things to do" to avoid real intimacy with one another. These two problems would be the main focus of the family therapy.

Over the following eight weeks of family therapy, we made observations about the difficulties the family had in accomplishing tasks they set for themselves because they did not attend to the emotional aspects of their relationships. A simple example of this involved the purchase of a pair of swimming flippers for Mark by his father. Mark reported that he was in a "bad mood" and did not feel like buying flippers, but that his father insisted on doing it because it was a convenient time to do so. The result was that the flippers didn't fit and that both father and son were angry and hurt.

We suggested family projects; some that had a task focus and some that had an emotional focus. It became clear fairly quickly that the tasks involving working on emotional issues were not accomplished, whereas those with a clear, concrete goal—such as making a star chart for good behaviors—were more easily and readily completed. Gently discussing this trend with the family was enough for them to see that their perception of limited time might not be the entire reason for why the family was not doing well and why Mark's eating problems persisted.

The family's strengths were built on as much as possible, and we initiated a star chart to assist Mark with eating. The star chart rewarded normal eating patterns; no rewards were generated for Mark's maladaptive eating patterns. Mark established what he wanted to earn and the specifics of what foods would be included on the chart. The major difficulty with the star chart was, predictably, that the family didn't keep it up. As with any behavioral system, reinforcement of positive behaviors must be immediate and consistent. What made it difficult for Mark's family to maintain the star chart was not a lack of intellectual understanding or willingness to comply but rather a family dynamic that allowed no one to really depend on other family members for emotional support.

INDIVIDUAL THERAPY

Prior to starting therapy, Mark had clearly established the cognitive ability to act and play in ways that expressed much about other situations that were occurring in his life. However, this capability was overwhelmed by his need for stable parental figures who would provide emotional care. Mark's mother reported that he had significant problems with separation from her that had begun at an early age. She reported that when she attempted to place him in a nursery school, he threw tantrums to prevent her from leaving. This behavior continued until he started second grade, when he suddenly stopped; he told her "Other children don't have their mothers here" and sent her away. It was shortly after this incident that his sister was born. His restrictive eating patterns emerged within this context.

In Mark's individual play therapy, he developed a play world in which his needs were better addressed. In that world, he created characters who protected him and were available to help him in his various "crusades." The major themes of Mark's play therapy were associated with insecurity and fear of abandonment. His managed his own neediness in a "counterphobic" way by identifying in his play with powerful and magical figures. We encouraged his use of fantasy to help him manage his feelings of dependency. To children, play is "real" in that it allows them to work through their emotional problems in an age-appropriate manner. It is not important that a school-age child abstractly understand that he is playing at being an all-powerful wizard in order to compensate for feeling anxious and dependent. What is important is that the play be effective—that is, that it promotes a change in the child's feelings. Prior to starting play therapy, Mark was unable to play effectively in this sense.

In order to help Mark elaborate on themes in his play, we made comments on how a character seemed to be acting or feeling. For example, if Mark was playing with a magic sorcerer, we would say, "It looks like the sorcerer is powerful, and happy being able to do these magical things." Mark might not respond verbally but would pick up on this theme and have the sorcerer become even more powerful and happier with himself. Another technique we used was to comment indirectly on the possible meaning of some part of the play. Mark might have one of his knights killing an evil villain, and we would comment, "Sometimes boys feel so angry at not getting their way they feel like hurting someone, maybe even someone they love." This type of statement usually came after rapport and play were well established. Comments such as these directed the play toward more personal themes. In this case, Mark made the knight seek out another knight with whom to fight over a princess. The play was now less distant from his real competitive strivings with his brother and father for his mother's love and attention.

In addition to the problems already discussed, Mark had difficulty with expected gender role behaviors with his peers. He was considered a "nerd" and a "wimp." His older brother persecuted him about these "weaknesses" as well. Mark had no problem with being a boy, but he did feel uncomfortable with overt aggressive feelings and actions. Much of this was linked to an unconscious fear of his controlling father and much was projected onto his imperious older brother. Overt fighting between the boys was a constant problem. However, Mark had to carefully gauge his fighting, as he was at a decided physical disadvantage. He was able to express aggression in his play, but still he expressed a fair amount of discomfort when the possibility of even symbolic self-injury occurred.

BEHAVIORAL INTERVENTION

The behavioral therapies that we use with school-age children with eating disorders are based on identifying and preventing eating-disordered behaviors and rewarding their interruption. With a school-age child, the concrete rewards of a star chart or point system are effective. As in Mark's case, though, families with chaotic structures often have difficulty maintaining a reward system, and it is likely that they will require much assistance from you. Also, we have found that eating disordered behaviors can serve to "soothe" children; by helping the child find alternatives for self-soothing, you will assist her in giving up the behaviors.

RESOLUTION

Mark's fear of abandonment and his separation anxiety, frustrated anger, and suppression of intimate feelings ultimately led to eating problems. In his mind, by regulating what he ate he could control his neediness and be satisfied on his own terms. Over the course of several months of family, individual, and behavioral therapy, the family began to express emotions more readily, and Mark was more confident that his own needs would be met. He was able to use fantasy and play as an age-appropriate way to manage what he could not control; he no longer required the "action language" of not eating to "repeat" his problems over and over, and his atypical eating behaviors ceased.

Medical Treatment

The health of school-age children with eating disorders is likely to deteriorate rapidly. These children often exhibit more rapid weight loss and need more immediate medical attention than adolescents or adults with eating disorders.

Nutritional Education. We work with a nutritionist on our team who provides nutritional education to children and their families. If you work with school-age children with eating disorders, it is important to decide on a case-by-case basis whether you need to involve a professional nutritionist. It usually is not necessary to involve a nutritionist in cases where the eating problem is secondary to trauma or is without medical complications. In other cases, we recommend at least an initial consultation with someone to educate the family about the consequences, from a nutritional perspective, of the child's current behaviors. The nutritionist can often also educate pediatricians on these matters. In cases involving children with severe and chronic eating disorders, a nutritionist, along with the pediatrician, can act as a "reality check" on a child's progress.

Medical Monitoring. School-age children with eating disorders that are severe enough to have medical consequences—usually involving severe weight loss or chronic vomiting—should have scheduled visits with their pediatricians to make sure that they are medically stable enough to stay in outpatient treatment. Children who lose too much weight or who fail to gain adequate weight are at risk for severe problems with their hearts and bones. When we start work with such children, we ask that they visit their pediatricians sometimes up to twice a week for checkups. As children begin to get a handle on their problems, these visits can be cut back. We do not recommend starting treatment of a child with a suspected eating disorder unless a pediatrician is involved in the care.

Related Therapeutic Issues

As you work with the treatments that we have discussed, you will likely come across issues related to the therapeutic process and the context in which the treatment is taking place.

Countertransference. When working with children and families with eating disorders, you should be alert to countertransference issues. It has sometimes been hard for us to develop empathy for a child who is so bent on self-destructive behaviors. These children are often very unavailable emotionally, and this can make it difficult to connect with them. One young doctor in training discussed with us how bored she was working with children with Anorexia Nervosa. She said their personalities seemed to her like what Gertrude Stein said about Oakland, California: "There's no there, there." The doctor's boredom reflected a much deeper hostility toward these young children, and her quotation suggested a wish to make them "not there."

On the other hand, children with purging and bingeing disorders have often appeared to us as emotionally labile and very needy. We sometimes intuitively respond to these children by developing "rescue fantasies" that make it difficult to work with the family in a productive way. We may also react negatively to this emotional lability and neediness by withdrawing from the child. We must be alert to these developments in ourselves and seek assistance from supervisors or consultants when they occur.

Managed Care. We live in a time of managed health care resources. All of us know this means we need to do more with less. Children are often treated as second-class citizens in managed care systems. This is true, in part, because parents and their companies purchase health care plans oriented toward adult care. What this means for children is that they often do not have the same access to care—especially mental health care—as adults do.

For children with eating disorders, the problems are more complicated, because, as we have described, they often require treatment from a variety of persons—all of whom cost the managed care system money. When a child with an eating disorder is referred to us, we discuss the overall treatment plan and its rationale with the reviewer who will be certifying the visits. We emphasize the importance of aggressive early care and the need for a multidisciplinary approach. We ask the pediatrician, who is sometimes the gatekeeper to the mental health portions of a plan, to advocate for this approach. This requires education of the pediatrician at times, and always involves continuing work with reviewers. We also ask families to take whatever responsibility they can for the type of health care plan they have chosen and to recognize that they may need to pay for some services out of pocket. Overall, our experience with managed care is not unlike our experience with other health care providers—a lot depends on the particular company you're dealing with and how you approach them.

PREVENTION

Treatment of eating disorders can be successful, but as with any type of problem, we ideally want to prevent the symptoms from occurring in the first place. Unfortunately, studies show that prevention programs for adolescents and adults have resulted in only minimal changes in weight-related attitudes and weight-loss behaviors. One reason for this might be that by attacking these problems in adolescence and adulthood, the intervention comes too late. Linda Smolak and Michael Levine argue convincingly for the use of prevention programs with elementary school children.

It is during the school-age years that significant factors can be recognized and dealt with before they have a chance to greatly influence the child's development. Take the time to identify early risk factors and to work with at-risk individuals before it's too late. In some cases, basic information will be all that is necessary to prevent later problems. However, other young people may need you to work closely and individually with them.

Working with school-age children to prevent and treat eating disorders can be exceptionally rewarding. These young people can really benefit from your help. They are fairly articulate about their problems and work with you to establish a healthy foundation on which to venture into adolescence. Your input at this young age can allow for the development of positive attributes that will last a lifetime. Just imagine the prospect of empowering young children to find healthy ways to cope; to feel good about their bodies; and to stay away from starving, bingeing, purging, and all of the other unhealthy behaviors that accompany eating disorders. In our work with school-age children, we have seen children steered away from the all-too-common problems of body dissatisfaction and unhealthy eating. To have played some part in allowing them to gain a sense of competence and to experience life without constantly worrying about their weight and their eating is extremely rewarding.

NOTES

P. 217, *Anorexia Nervosa occurs less than 10 percent of the time in children under the age of eleven:* Lucas, A. R., Beard, C. M., O'Fallow, W. M., & Karland, L. T. (1991). 50 year trends in the incidence of anorexia nervosa in Rochester, Minnesota: A population-based study. *American Journal of Psychiatry, 148,* 917–922.

P. 217, *subclinical concerns regarding weight and dieting occur in close to 50 percent of school-age girls:* Maloney, M. J., McGuire, J., Daniels, S. R., & Specker, B. (1989). Dieting behavior and eating attitudes in children. *Pediatrics, 84*(3), 482–488.

P. 218, *One study found that 45 percent of third through sixth graders:* Maloney, M. J., McGuire, J., Daniels, S. R., & Specker, B. (1989). *ibid.,* pp. 482–487.

P. 218, *a link between fourth- and fifth-grade girls' weight concerns:* Taylor, C. B., Altman, T., Shisslak, C., Bryson, S., Estes, L. S., Gray, N., McKnight, K. M., Kraemer, H. C., & Killen, J. D. (in press). Factors associated with weight concerns in adolescents. *International Journal of Eating Disorders.*

P. 218, *girls outnumber boys approximately ten to one with regard to developing eating disorders:* Hsu, L. G. (1989). The gender gap in eating disorders: Why are the eating disorders more common among women? *Clinical Psychology Review, 9*(3), 393–407.

P. 218, *more equally distributed among school-age boys and girls:* Fosson, A., Knibbs, J., Bryant-Waugh, R., & Lask, B. (1987). Early onset anorexia nervosa. *Archives of Disease in Childhood, 62,* 114–118.

P. 218, *Other biological factors that are not considered here:* Steiner, H., Sanders, M., & Ryst, E. (1995). Precursors and risk factors of juvenile eating disorders. In H. C. Steinhausen (Ed.), *Eating disorders in adolescence.* Hawthorne, NY: Walter de Gruyter.

P. 218, *More than 90 percent of anorectics and 80 percent of bulimics are female:* Casper, R. C., & Offer, D. (1990). Weight and dieting concerns in adolescents: Fashion or symptom? *Pediatrics, 86,* 384–390.

P. 219, *Puberty (especially early onset of puberty) may be a risk factor:* Killen, J. D., Hayward, C., Litt, I., Hammer, L. D., Wilson, D. M., Miner, B., Taylor, C. B., Varady, A., & Shisslak, C. (1992). Is puberty a risk factor for eating disorders? *American Journal of Diseases in Children, 146,* 323–325.

P. 220, *Excessive weight concern predicts the onset of eating disorders:* Killen, J. D., Taylor, C. B., Hayward, C., Wilson, D. M., Haydel, K. F., Hammer, L. D., Simmonds, B., Robinson, T. N., Litt, I., Varady, A., & Kraemer, H. (1994). The pursuit of thinness and onset of eating disorder symptoms in a community sample of adolescent girls: A three-year prospective analysis. *International Journal of Eating Disorders, 16,* 227–238; Killen, J. D., Taylor, C. B., Hayward, C., Haydel, K. F., Wilson, D. M., Hammer, L. D., Kraemer, H., Blair-Greiner, A., & Strachowski, D. (in press). Weight concerns influence the development of eating disorders: A four-year prospective study. *Journal of Consulting and Clinical Psychology.*

P. 220, *By age thirteen, 80 percent of girls have already been on a weight-loss diet:* Mellin, L. M., Scully, S., & Irving, C. E. (1986). *Disordered eating characteristics in preadolescent girls.* Paper presented at the annual meeting of the American Dietetic Association, Las Vegas, NV.

P. 220, *they can often be compliant, perfectionistic, . . . and sometimes obsessive:* Steiner, H., Sanders, M., & Ryst, E. (1995). *ibid.*

P. 222, *The level of family disturbance is often high:* DiNicola, V. F., Roberts, N., & Oke, L. (1989). Eating and mood disorders in young children. *Psychiatric Clinics of North America, 12*(4), 873–893.

P. 222, *When a parent is preoccupied with his or her own thinness and food intake:* Hill, A. J., Weaver, C., & Blundell, J. E. (1990). Dieting concerns of 10-year-old girls and their mothers. *British Journal of Clinical Psychology, 29,* 346–348.

P. 223, *School-age children with eating problems and weight concerns are . . . about their relationships:* Altman, T. M., Killen, J. D., Bryson, S. W.,

Shisslak, C. M., Estes, L. S., McKnight, K. M., Gray, N., Crago, M., & Taylor, C. B. (in press). Attachment style and weight concerns in preadolescent and adolescent girls. *International Journal of Eating Disorders.*

P. 225, *The* DSM-IV *lists the following criteria for Anorexia Nervosa:* American Psychiatric Association. (1994). *Diagnostic and statistical manual of mental disorders* (4th ed., pp. 539–550). Washington, DC: Author.

P. 239, *studies show that prevention programs for adolescents and adults have resulted in only minimal changes:* Taylor, C. B., & Altman, T. (1996). *Priorities in prevention research for eating disorders.* Manuscript submitted for publication.

P. 239, *Linda Smolak and Michael Levine argue convincingly:* Smolak, L., & Levine, M. P. (1994). Toward an empirical basis for primary prevention of eating problems with elementary school children. *Eating Disorders, 2*(4), 293–307.

ABOUT THE AUTHORS

Tamara M. Altman, B.A., is researcher in the Department of Psychiatry and Behavioral Sciences at Stanford University School of Medicine. She earned her B.A. degree in psychology at the University of California at Berkeley. She is currently the project director of a longitudinal, multisite study involving the identification of risk factors for the development of eating disorders in young girls. Her research and publications have focused on weight concerns, eating disorders, attachment styles, and stress and coping of children and adolescents.

Pamela J. Beasley, M.D., earned her B.A. from the University of Pennsylvania and her M.D. from the Hahnemann University School of Medicine. She is a child psychiatrist and director of the consultation-liaison service in the Department of Psychiatry at Children's Hospital and is instructor in psychiatry at Harvard Medical School in Boston.

Lisa R. Benton-Hardy, M.D., is chief fellow in child and adolescent psychiatry, Division of Child Psychiatry and Development at the Stanford University School of Medicine. As a scholar at the Violence Prevention Initiative Program of The California Wellness Foundation at Stanford University, she has worked with children who have been exposed to violence and who have developed the complete spectrum of psychiatric disorders. She received the Presidential Scholar Award in the category of research from the American Academy of Child and Adolescent Psychiatry in 1996. Her other interests include working with youth from diverse cultural and socioeconomic backgrounds.

Julie A. Collier, Ph.D., is clinical instructor in the Department of Psychiatry and Behavioral Sciences at Stanford University School of Medicine, and program director of the pediatric psychiatry consultation-liaison service at Lucile Salter Packard

Children's Hospital at Stanford. Her clinical and research interests include coping with chronic illness, psychological trauma related to medical treatment, somatization, and psychological issues associated with pediatric organ transplants.

David Ray DeMaso, M.D., earned his B.S. and M.D. from the University of Michigan. He is a child psychiatrist and clinical director of the Department of Psychiatry at Children's Hospital, and is associate professor of psychiatry at Harvard Medical School in Boston.

Jennifer Dyer-Friedman, Ph.D., received her Ph.D. in clinical psychology from the University of California at Berkeley. She is a postdoctoral fellow in the Division of Child Psychiatry and Development at Stanford University School of Medicine. Dr. Dyer-Friedman's clinical interests are in the treatment of adolescents and their families. Her research interests are in bridging clinical practice and research through the development of new methods clinicians can use to assess and describe their adolescent and adult patients.

S. Shirley Feldman, Ph.D., obtained her B.A. in Melbourne, Australia, and her Ph.D. in developmental psychology from Stanford University. She has taught at Stanford University for the last twenty-five years and served as director of the Stanford Center for the Study of Families, Children, and Youth for four years (1991–1995). She has done extensive research and writing on the socialization of children and adolescents and has conducted longitudinal studies spanning the transitions from childhood into early adolescence and from late adolescence into adulthood.

James Lock, Ph.D., M.D., is an assistant professor of child psychiatry in the Department of Psychiatry and Behavioral Sciences at Stanford University School of Medicine, and medical director of the comprehensive pediatric care unit at the Lucile Salter Packard Children's Hospital at Stanford. He received his Ph.D.

from Emory University and his M.D. from Morehouse School of Medicine.

Dr. Lock's main research activities have focused on the treatment of depression, eating disorders, and sexual development in children and adolescents. He has published articles on psychotherapeutic treatment of eating disorders, Attention Deficit Hyperactivity Disorder, and sexual development.

Zakee Matthews, M.D., obtained his M.D. from the University of Missouri, Columbia. In 1993, he was selected as an Academic Scholar of The California Wellness Foundation Violence Prevention Initiative at Stanford University. In 1992, he received the Presidential Scholars Award of the American Academy of Child and Adolescent Psychiatry in the category Public Policy. Currently, he is clinical instructor and medical director of the Adolescent Alcohol and Substance Abuse Program in the Division of Child Psychiatry and Development at the Stanford University School of Medicine. Dr. Matthews's research interests encompass childhood trauma, substance abuse, and juvenile delinquency.

Mary J. Sanders, Ph.D., received her Ph.D. in clinical psychology from Memphis State University. She is the director of psychological services and is clinical instructor in the Division of Child Psychiatry and Development at Stanford University School of Medicine. Dr. Sanders has worked in the field of child abuse for the past twenty years. Since 1986, she has been at Lucile Salter Packard Children's Hospital at Stanford, where she is a specialist in the areas of child abuse and eating disorders.

Richard J. Shaw, M.B., B.S., is assistant professor in the Division of Child Psychiatry at Stanford University School of Medicine. He is also medical director of consultation-liaison services at Lucile Salter Packard Children's Hospital at Stanford. Dr. Shaw is a native of Zimbabwe and a graduate of Middlesex Hospital Medical School, University of London, England. His research interests include the study of affect expression and affect recognition in schizophrenia, and more recently the study of adjustment in children with severe medical illnesses.

Hans Steiner, M.D., is professor of psychiatry and behavioral sciences in the Division of Child Psychiatry and Development at the Stanford University School of Medicine. He is a fellow of the American Psychiatric Association, the American Academy of Child and Adolescent Psychiatry, and the Academy of Psychosomatic Medicine.

Dr. Steiner has received the Outstanding Mentor Award of the American Academy of Child and Adolescent Psychiatry in 1990, 1992, 1993, 1995, and 1996. He also received the Dlin/Fischer Award for significant achievement in clinical research by the Academy of Psychosomatic Medicine in 1993. In 1994, he was selected by *Good Housekeeping* as one of the nation's 327 best mental health care providers. In 1996, the American Medical Association awarded him the Joseph B. Goldberger Award for his clinical work and research in eating disorders.

Dr. Steiner is a native of Austria and a graduate of the Vienna University Faculty of Medicine. His research and clinical work is concentrated on the adolescent age group. He is an internationally known expert on eating disorders, trauma-related psychopathology, and juvenile delinquency, and he lectures widely in Europe, Asia, and the United States.

Sharon E. Williams, Ph.D., is a postdoctoral fellow in child psychology in the Division of Child Psychiatry and Development at the Stanford University School of Medicine. She received her Ph.D. in clinical psychology from the University of Cincinnati. Dr. Williams is an Academic fellow with The California Wellness Foundation; she conducts violence-related research under the foundation's Violence Prevention Initiative. Her clinical interests include working with children who have been abused or otherwise traumatized and those exposed to violence. Her research interests include the effects of abuse and violence on youth, particularly female youth. Her current research investigates factors that influence adolescent dating violence.

INDEX